Superskin

Superskin

Natural Ways to Super Healthy Skin

Kathryn Marsden

Thorsons

Thorsons
An Imprint of HarperCollins*Publishers*
77–85 Fulham Palace Road,
Hammersmith, London W6 8JB

The Thorsons website address is: www.thorsons.com

and *Thorsons* are trademarks of HarperCollins*Publishers* Limited

First published by Thorsons 1993
This edition published by Thorsons 2002

10 9 8 7 6 5 4 3 2 1

© Kathryn Marsden 1993, 2002

Kathryn Marsden asserts the moral right to
be identified as the author of this work

A catalogue record for this book
is available from the British Library

ISBN 0 00 713298 0

Printed and bound in Great Britain by
Martins the Printers Limited, Berwick-upon-Tweed

About the Author

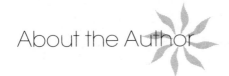

Kathryn Marsden is the author of more than a dozen books, including the phenomenal best-sellers *The Food Combining Diet*, *Food Combining in 30 Days* and *The Complete Book of Food Combining*. Her inspiration for *Super Skin* came from years of misery and depression caused by skin problems which doctors could not resolve. As a result of her own research into nutrition and diet, and her personal success against huge odds in restoring her own complexion to glowing good health, she is a true inspiration to others. A nutritionist with over a decade of practitioner experience, Kathryn has written extensively on health and beauty for national newspapers and for leading glossies both in the UK and overseas. She believes passionately that, whilst ageing is inevitable, beauty is achievable at any age. And has proved it!

Kathryn is a fabulous 50-something who is known for her wacky sense of humour, her loyalty to her friends and her generosity of spirit. She is an impassioned gardener and a devotee of organic food who is wild about wildlife and her gorgeous husband, Richard. She lives among 'some of the kindest people on the planet' in the Western Isles of Scotland, where she has escaped to work on her next book.

Kathryn's views are completely independent. She is not employed by any skin care company, supplement supplier or food producer and is not paid or in any other way persuaded to recommend the products of any particular company.

The information that Kathryn includes in her books, feature articles and lectures has been accumulated from her own personal research and experience, which, from the feedback she has received, would appear to have helped many people. However, it is important that the reader understands that these guidelines are not intended to be prescriptive, nor are they an attempt to diagnose or treat any specific condition.

If you are concerned in any way about your health, Kathryn strongly recommends that you visit your general practitioner or hospital consultant without delay. She also suggests that you keep your medical adviser informed of any dietary changes and of any supplement programmes that you intend to follow. Obtain as many details as possible about your condition, asking plenty of questions about medicines which may be prescribed to you. Do not stop taking any currently prescribed medicines without first talking to your doctor. In the meantime, follow a varied and sensible diet made up of fresh, unprocessed wholefoods, two pieces of fresh fruit, two or three servings of fresh vegetables and a salad each day, plus at least four glasses of filtered or bottled water. Take regular exercise and avoid cigarette smoke.

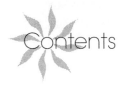

Contents

Foreword by Katie Boyle

After the runaway success of Kathryn Marsden's book *The Food Combining Diet*, I reached out eagerly for her next publication. I wasn't disappointed. The Marsden Magic was there again: real knowledge of her subject, combined with sensible solutions to the problems she tackles.

I feel so safe in Kathryn Marsden's hands and her direct style makes her advice very easy to follow.

KATIE BOYLE, LONDON 1994

This updated version – of what was an already pretty comprehensive book – is a joy. Existing chapters are expanded and there's so much that's new and interesting. Kathryn helps us to choose and use essential oils, looks at nutritious and delicious skin foods and explains the benefits of eating organically. We learn how stress can play havoc with our skin – and what we can do about it; also how to detox safely and, something most of us don't do well, how to breathe properly. No preaching, just plenty of wisdom. If ever a book could be called a 'treasure chest' and a perfect size for bedtime reading, I believe this is it.

KATIE BOYLE, LONDON 2002

> To help you make the best of your skin, Kathryn Marsden's *Super Skin* is packed with helpful and healthful beauty tips, advice on diet, hair and nail care, nutritional supplements, first aid for particular problems and how to detoxify and cleanse the system – all designed to get you glowing.

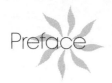
Preface

We are responsible for our own beauty and well-being in all our relationships. To create this, we need a good balance of diet, exercise and relaxation to heal our body and soul. Nature radiates its own life force, promoting healing and a sense of wellbeing which we can tap into. Thus we can heal ourselves on many levels, give back what we have taken and endeavour to co-exist harmoniously.

DR JURGEN KLEIN

NATUROPATH AND BIOCHEMIST

FOUNDER OF JURLIQUE INTERNATIONAL

This book is for anyone who cares about their skin, whether that means that they have a particular skin problem, are bothered by a dry, oily, flaky, dull or blemished complexion or are simply in need of care and attention. Whether you're young or older, troubled by teenage acne or worried about wrinkles or the unavoidable fact that *tempus fugit* (literally, 'time flies'), then this book is for you, too.

Skin problems can make life a misery. I know: I speak from irksome experience. From the onset of periods at age 14, I began my fight against the dreaded zits. 'There, there, you'll grow out of it' and sympathetic head-patting from dermatologists, doctors and relatives did absolutely nothing to make me feel better.

Long and arduous visits to a number of hospitals and a variety of different specialists eventually detected a serious endocrine disorder ('probably inherited') which, it was felt, 'might' ('or might not') be causing or aggravating the skin problem. A whole gamut of medical tests resulted in two major operations which eased the hormonal horrors – but the eruptions persisted.

Could it be my diet? *'What you eat will make no difference whatsoever to the condition of your skin'* I was – so I thought – reliably informed. And 30 years on, a leaflet to be found in many a doctor's waiting room continues to maintain that what a person eats will have neither beneficial nor detrimental effect upon their skin condition. 'There is no scientific evidence that chocolate or fatty foods contribute to the problem,' it proclaims.

If it wasn't diet, then it must surely have something to do with what I put on the outside. An allergy, a reaction to something that I wasn't yet aware of? So I gave up on the food thing and turned my attention to any lotion or cream that might help from the outside. Despite copious and diligent application, nothing I bought made much difference, perhaps drying up a few existing spots but doing zilch to prevent new ones from forming. Over-enthusiastic dedication to very strong-smelling chemical astringents (you'll try anything when you're desperate) and some strange white paint-like substance from the doctor only made matters worse, adding dry, sore and flaky skin to the ever-present blemishes and leaving me with red blotches and scarring.

And they wondered why I was a depressed teenager.

Perhaps, after all, I would just have to wait to grow out of it.

On reaching the milestone of 21, I was convinced that I would soon be spot-free. No such luck.

'Growing out of it' was obviously not going to happen to me.

But then something happened in my life that brought about a change of diet. Within six months of making those changes, my skin had improved enormously. Its condition now bears no comparison to the angry, sore appearance that I suffered – and tried in vain to hide – for so many years.

Because of the previously over-aggressive treatments, I didn't believe my skin would ever be perfect, but over the years even the deep blemishes, which I was told would always be there, have faded. So different is it now that a student at one of my nutrition lectures asked me recently if I would mind telling the class what type of make-up I use because my skin 'looks so smooth and firm'. My honest answer was 'none'. Just a great diet, good quality moisturizers and regular exercise.

Now, if what the medical establishment says about diet having no effect on the resolution of skin disorders is true, how is it that I – and many others – have managed to attain a good complexion by changing our eating habits?

For me, diet definitely does work. I have absolutely no doubt that it was – and is – the stimulus that made the difference; that the wrong kinds of foods can really 'upset' the skin, while the right ones have the power to heal.

A good example is chocolate. I have had patients who swear that one piece of chocolate equals one spot. Well, in my experience as a spot-ridden teenager turned clear-skinned nutritionist, I agree with them. Just show me a box of chocolates and zits appear overnight. My only regret is that it took so many years for me to discover that the 'experts' might not have all the answers.

Treating the surface symptoms – the dryness, the blemishes, the eczema, etc. is all very well, but does nothing to discover or resolve the cause of the condition.

Experience has shown me that the way to success is to treat the whole body, inside and out, *naturally*: super skin foods supported by a top quality cleansing and nourishing routine, lots of refreshing sleep, regular exercise and a little help from alternative remedies such as good vitamin supplements, herbal remedies and essential oils. And you'll find them all here, in *Superskin*.

Need More Help?

Superskin contains lots of good advice for all skin types and for many different skin problems. But I'm obviously not going to be able to answer all your questions. If you have a particular skin problem which needs special attention or you simply need extra help, why not treat yourself to a personal consultation with a qualified beauty therapist or facialist?

❋ Choose someone with an established reputation who has been recommended. Word of mouth is the way you hear about both the good and the ghastly.

⁕ Book an appointment for a facial, but try to time it so it's not around PMS or period week.

⁕ Before you book, ask about cost, how long you need to be there and what is involved. Ask about the training and experience of the practitioner who is going to look after you.

⁕ Once there, you should be given the opportunity to discuss the treatment before it begins and have time to tell the therapist about any particular skin problems you may have.

⁕ I'd be very cautious if anti-comedome (blackhead-removing) tools are suggested. I was treated with these in the past and found that, although they unblocked the pores, they left minor scarring instead.

⁕ Ask your therapist to talk you through the treatment as he or she progresses. It's reassuring to know what's coming next and what products are being used.

⁕ When you've found someone you like and trust, go as regularly as you can afford. Look upon good skin care as a necessary luxury.

If you're just unsure about your skin type and feel that you'd like to update the skin care products you use (we should all do this regularly, especially as we grow older), then the beauty pages of women's magazines can be a useful source of information. Or you may consider asking advice from a beauty counter consultant in one of the larger chemists or department stores.

⁕ Don't restrict your questions to one counter. Talk to as many as possible; it could help you to sort the sales hype from the worthwhile guidance.

⁕ Remember that, however helpful your consultant is, she is there to sell her company's products!

⁕ If you're unsure, ask for samples to try before you buy, and don't be persuaded to purchase lots of full-sized expensive jars or bottles which may be unsuitable. If you even suspect that you won't use a product, don't be pressurized into buying it.

⁂ Don't be afraid to say 'no'; if it's not what you are looking for or it's beyond your budget, don't hang around.

⁂ Although there are lots of great products which can make a definite difference to skin health and condition, you don't need a drawer-full.

⁂ Never fall for the sales pitch that one product won't work unless it is used in conjunction with another – it's unlikely to be true.

While I was researching for this book, I talked to consultants from all the major skin-care and cosmetic companies. Some were excellent; some, well, not so ... I have to say that the range of advice can be confusing; which just goes to show that the 'experts' all have individual ideas and views on how to achieve perfect skin and every person has utterly individual requirements.

In the space of one week, different experts told me I had oily, combination, sensitive, not sensitive and dry skin. I should exfoliate more often; I should exfoliate less often; I should use a special eye cleanser; no, that wasn't necessary, as my ordinary cleanser was adequate, etc., etc. I also enjoyed several make-up sessions, although I found most a bit heavy-handed. Some colours looked stunning and others, oh woe ... a few of the consultants' ideas on which colours suited me were so way off the mark that several friends wondered if I was quite well ... loaded eye liner and foundation (which I rarely wear), brown and purple shadows, overemphasized blusher and dark lipstick conspired to make a healthy nutritionist look tired and consumptive!

At the end of it all, I was able to take the best bits of advice from all the sources I had consulted and put them together in a package to suit my personal needs. These days, that tends to include natural skin care – using products made using as-natural-as-possible ingredients, rather than laboratory-produced chemicals – and only gentle make-up for eyes, cheeks and lips.

And can I say, finally, that I am not a skin specialist or a beautician and would not wish, in any way, to denigrate those professionals. I'm a nutritionist with a passionate interest in natural skin care. I write purely from my own experience – and that of my patients – through which I hope to show you the natural way to a clear, glowing and healthy complexion.

I have always wanted to write a book about skin health to record my own observations so that they might help others. Some of the tips included may not toe the orthodox line, but they are gentle, entirely safe and, most important of all, they work.

I hope they help you, too.

Wishing you always the best of health.

KATHRYN MARSDEN

P.S. As far as my extensive research can confirm, none of the methods or products mentioned in the book has caused harm to any animal. Animals don't wear cosmetics. Because we do, why should they suffer?

Introduction: The Superskin Strategy

Looking Good

Appearances do matter. Looking good makes people feel good. Looking
after yourself and your skin makes very good sense. How you look projects
your personality and demonstrates that you're thinking positively about
yourself.

For the young, looking good becomes all-important – for some, a consuming passion. But someone with not-so-great skin may feel there's little
point in bothering, especially if they've already tried to resolve their problems
without success. And for many more, as the years advance, interest in hair
care, skin care, make-up, healthy eating, posture and dress begins to wane.

It shouldn't have to and doesn't need to.

I'm convinced that lots of very lovely people never reach their full
potential simply because they hide themselves and their inner beauty
underneath shapeless, colourless clothing, dull, lifeless hair, a boring,
flavourless and nutrient-deficient diet and dated or non-existent make-up.
No wonder they feel depressed, tired and lacking in self-esteem.

There are bound to be people reading this who disagree with me.
'Bah! Humbug!' they will say. 'It doesn't matter what someone looks like.
It's the actual person that's important. Inner beauty will shine through no
matter what.'

Of course it can. But what's wrong with giving it a little encourage-
ment? After all, how a person looks is often a reflection of how they feel.
And feelings affect attitude.

Cosmetic beauty may be only skin-deep, but real beauty reflects your
whole being. And the two *are* connected. I believe that there is an inextricable

link between good health and beauty at all levels. Good skin care and hair care can transform a personality. Even something as simple as applying some lipstick or giving your nails a salon treatment can chase a negative outlook away for long enough to spur you into more positive action.

Nourishing and nurturing yourself properly bring immense and immeasurable rewards of confidence, vitality, energy, positiveness and good health, of looking and feeling good – inside and out.

And age really has nothing to do with it. One person's wrinkle is merely another person's laughter line.

⚘ Your Skin and How It Functions

Skin is an amazing structure. The body's largest organ, covering between 1.5 and 2 square metres (15 and 20 square feet), it measures a tenth of a millimetre thick (one-twentieth of an inch) and weighs anything from 2.75 to 4 kilograms (6 to 9 pounds). This wonderful 'waterproof' and washable coat serves as a temperature regulator, a major route for the elimination of waste and, given the right nutrients, has the incredible capacity to heal itself when injured and act as an efficient defence against trauma, infection and invasion. 'Like a wax paper that holds everything in without dripping' is how skin was once described by the US television personality with the wonderful name Art Linkletter.

Healthy skin is slightly acid and is protected by the 'acid mantle', a naturally lubricating mixture of sebum and sweat which provides additional protection against assault by harmful bacteria. The skin and its padding also cushion internal organs against impact.

Through approximately two and a half million sweat glands, the average adult human being loses around 850 millilitres (a pint and a half) of sweat each day. In every square inch there are hundreds of pain, heat, cold and touch sensors, 5 metres (15 feet) of blood vessels, 4 metres (12 feet) of nerves, 100 sebaceous glands and over 1,500 sensory receptors, totalling three million cells, all shedding constantly – at an amount equal to an entire layer every seven to ten weeks.

This perpetual 'moulting' means that, to maintain the status quo, new cells need to be formed at an equivalent rate.

The outer surface (the epidermis) is actually a layer of dead keratin cells which are continually being shed and replaced by new cells working their way up from the dermis below. When this exfoliation process becomes sluggish – as we grow older or when health is under par – cell renewal slows right down, elimination pathways can become blocked, skin is less supple and so becomes more prone to injury and disease.

To remain in good condition and to work efficiently, your birthday suit needs to be fed and cleaned from the inside as well as the outside.

Superskin shows you how easy it is to achieve that fresh, vital visage:

The Superskin Four-point Protection Plan

1   Diet and Nutrition: Healthy skin depends on a healthy diet brimful of healing and nurturing nutrients. *Superskin* gives you the food facts on what's good – and not so good – for your skin type.

2   Detox: A regular one- or two-day detox diet, using cleansing skin foods and purifying fluids, improves your beauty routine from the inside out, helping to clean up internal sludge, encourage efficient elimination of wastes and re-energize your system.

3   Beauty on the Outside: It's just as important to take time to pamper yourself and attend to the external care of your skin – deep cleansing, exfoliation, massage, toning and moisturizing. You'll find some delicious home-made skin care remedies and plenty of natural-as-possible product recommendations.

4   Well-being: Stress, poor quality sleep, shallow breathing, inadequate exercise? They're all seriously bad for your skin and do nothing for your long term well-being. This book includes some easy-to-follow ideas on the best ways to relax, exercise, sleep and breathe to beat a stressful, exhausting world.

In many ways, ignoring any one of these important areas is a bit like expecting a four-legged table to stand firmly on only three legs. Without support at all four corners, everything begins to slide and, eventually, crashes to the floor.

part 1
·············

Diet and Nutrition

chapter 1

Superskin Foods and the Importance of Fats

> *The disease ceases without the use of any kind of medicine, if only a proper way of living be adopted.* AETIOS (C. AD 535)

Everything you (do or don't) put in your mouth is likely to affect the quality of your skin.

A clogged, spotty complexion often betrays a diet high in fats and sugars, a history of constipation, kidneys that are not working at their best or poor lymphatic drainage; an ultra-sensitive skin may be the result of poor digestion and inadequate absorption; very dry, flaky skin may indicate deficiencies of essential fatty acids and vitamin E; skin that refuses to heal could be in need of vitamins A, B_6, C and zinc.

The amazing thing is that skins like these can be completely transformed by making simple but beneficial changes to the diet, eating foods in the right combinations, using a regular internal and external cleansing programme, taking the right supplements and making time for regular exercise.

Skin quality can also be affected by the external environment, by cigarette smoking (passive or direct), traffic fumes, malfunctioning air-conditioning systems, central heating, radiation, VDU screens (see page 206) and excessive sun exposure. Nourishing food and protective skin care can help here too, providing defence against infection, cell damage and premature ageing.

The right kinds of foods will keep your intestines free of clutter, encourage all your elimination processes to function efficiently and keep your blood clean and fed with nutrients.

✿ Superskin Foods

As if put there to increase our anguish, there will always be the gorgeous creature who seems to live on junk food and yet looks wonderful without any apparent effort – probably blessed with an amazingly efficient digestive and detox system which can handle all that rubbish.

For those of us who don't fall into this category, Nature's natural beauty foods are there to help us.

In their raw state, vegetables, fruits, sprouted grains, sprouted seeds and herbs are rich in nutrients and natural enzymes, so it is important to make sure that your diet contains at least some raw food every day. Many kinds of fresh fruits, vegetables, salads and herbs are sensational skin fixers. They help to renew and refurbish, providing protection against further damage. For example, lemon juice applied topically is cleansing and healing; taken as a drink or in food it clears and cleanses from the inside out. Grapes, fresh pineapple, apples and kiwi fruits are wonderful skin foods. So are cabbage and vitamin A-rich carrots, beetroot and parsley. Botanicals such as artichoke, burdock, chelidonium, dandelion and sarsaparilla help to decongest the kidneys and liver, improving the outflow of waste products and taking the detox load off the overworked skin.

For the benefit of your skin – and your health – make full use of the healing sustenance provided by Mother Nature. All fruits, fresh salads and fresh vegetables will be of value; so are wholegrains, nuts, seeds, yoghurt, fresh fish – and fresh water! The skin foods detailed here are just some of the very best.

Fruits

Apples

Only around 40 calories and super-rich in vitamin C and that all-important soluble fibre called pectin, apples are essential in any detoxification and skin-healing programme. They're also useful for helping to stabilize cholesterol levels. The tartaric acid and malic acid content of apples helps to settle the digestion. To treat an upset stomach or diarrhoea, grate an apple and leave it exposed to the air for 15 minutes before eating. It seems that this is one of those rare instances where oxidation (browning) is therapeutic. Don't do this to fruit as a general rule, though! When slicing or grating apples for other purposes, always have fresh lemon juice handy to sprinkle over them – the lemon stops the apple from going brown. Apples are an excellent health tonic for the bowel and liver and apple juice a helpful remedy for the treatment of kidney stones and gallstones. The scent from a bowl of fresh apples is said to allay anxiety. Unfortunately, many fruit crops have become victims of over-zealous crop-spraying so, unless you know they are organic, it's best to discard the skins.

Apricots

Fresh or dried, apricots are loaded with beta-carotene and iron, both important skin nutrients. An excellent cleansing fruit. At times of illness – especially bronchitis, chest and throat infections, colds, catarrh or sinusitis – use a juicing machine or food processor to blend apricots into a soothing and nourishing drink. They are also reported to be beneficial in the treatment of constipation, intestinal parasites and gallstones. Try the familiar dried yellow apricots or the hard, round Hunza apricots. Washed thoroughly and soaked overnight, they make a wonderfully nourishing and sustaining start to the day. But avoid dried fruits that are sprayed with sulphur dioxide preservative and glazing agents: sulphites can cause skin rashes.

Bananas

I read recently that bananas should not be included in any cleansing diet because of their starch content. In fact, they are a rich source of potassium, vitamin A, vitamin C, iron, calcium, zinc, folic acid and pectin – all essential for healthy skin. Bananas are high in gentle but effective dietary fibre and are an excellent therapeutic for all kinds of bowel disorders – particularly constipation, haemorrhoids, colitis, irritable bowel and diarrhoea. An average-sized banana contains only 90 calories but is filling, sustaining and easy on the digestion – very useful as an energy boost between meals and especially helpful if you are trying to overcome 'chocoholism'. I see no reason whatsoever to exclude them.

Blackberries

A rich source of vitamin C. Very valuable as a blood-cleansing food, blackberries are recommended for the treatment of excess mucus – in catarrh, for example – and for constipation, anaemia, kidney problems, diarrhoea and menstrual cramps. An infusion made from blackberry leaves is wonderfully therapeutic for sore throats.

Blueberries

Well known for their antiseptic and blood-cleansing properties, blueberries can be helpful for anaemia, bowel problems, spots and blemishes and menstrual disorders. A good source of vitamins and minerals.

Figs

Fresh or dried, figs are packed with nourishment. Rich in calcium, iron and magnesium, dried figs are also one of the best fibre sources. Six dried figs and three glasses of water added daily to the diet is an excellent remedy for constipation. A sluggish bowel can be a common companion to sallow or spotty skin! Figs are also reported to be helpful in the treatment of Raynaud's syndrome, poor circulation, hypotension (low blood pressure), intestinal parasites and catarrh. The juice from soaked figs makes an excellent cough medicine and gargle for sore throats. Split open and soaked for five minutes in hand-hot water, fresh figs make a soothing poultice for boils and for abscesses of the skin or gums.

Grapefruit

Valuable for its fibre, pectin and vitamin C. The bioflavonoids found in the pith and skin segments are blood vessel-strengtheners, anti-inflammatory agents, powerful antioxidants and fighters of infection – all vital in the quest for healthy skin. An interesting point which I have noted with my own patients is that, whereas oranges and orange juice can aggravate arthritic conditions, fresh grapefruit seems to be helpful. Save grapefruit skin, grate and dry it and store in an airtight container; during the winter, use a teaspoon of the rind with equal quantities of mint, sage and dark honey as a soothing cold remedy.

Grapes

Eat as many as you like. Why not have a 'grape day' and eat nothing else? You'll munch your way through 3 lb (1.5 kg) or more, but shouldn't feel hungry. You'll rest your digestion, speed up the detox process and help your skin – all at the same time. Make sure that you wash the grapes really thoroughly. Drink plenty of filtered or spring water throughout the day, too – around 1.7 litres (3 pints).

Kiwi Fruit

Contain twice the vitamin C of an orange, around four times the fibre of a stick of celery and are a good source of vitamin E and potassium. A versatile fruit, wonderful for juicing and for packed lunches. Just cut in half and scoop the flesh from the skin with a teaspoon, or peel and slice.

Lemons

One of life's greatest cleansers, packed with vitamin C (twice that of oranges) and valuable bioflavonoids. Lemons are one of the top skin foods, cleansing, healing and protective of the delicate mucous membranes – the body's 'inside skin'. Wake up to a drink of hot water with a squeeze of fresh lemon juice. If you find the taste too sharp, then add a dribble of organic honey. Use boiled water, though, not water from the hot tap. And remember that lemon juice sold in bottles or in plastic imitation lemons will contain preservatives. An old remedy for wrinkles is to apply lemon juice directly to the skin, leave it for two or three hours and then massage with olive oil; this is also beneficial for the hands. A lemon juice-and-water rinse is good for dandruff and makes a cleansing mouthwash, especially helpful after a late night or an excess of alcohol when the inside of the mouth and throat feel 'unpleasant'. Rub lemon juice into the hands to remove stains, to heal cuts and to eliminate the odour of onions or fish.

Melons
It was once believed that melons were a waste of time from a nutritional point of view, because they are nearly 90 per cent water. Now we know that all melons are nourishing and cleansing, rich in vitamin C and potassium and a good source of folic acid, vitamin A and iron. Cantaloupe and watermelon are particularly valuable. Melons prefer to be eaten entirely on their own, not with any other kind of food: mixing them causes fermentation, digestive distress and poor absorption of nutrients. If you eat them as a starter, try to leave 15 minutes between courses.

Pineapple
Fresh pineapple contains some very useful enzymes and lots of vitamins and minerals; it's particularly rich in vitamin C and bromelain, both of which have anti-inflammatory properties. The heavier the pineapple, the more juice it is likely to contain. Canned pineapple (in its own juice) can be a useful standby but is far less nourishing than the fresh version.

Pumpkin
A very rich source of beta carotene, pumpkin makes a versatile addition to both sweet and savoury dishes. Reported to be beneficial in the treatment of fluid retention, low blood pressure, inflammation, ulceration, piles and varicose veins. Pumpkin seeds are an excellent skin food, being rich in

essential fatty acids. Also good for constipation and, when the seeds are made into a tea, for the elimination of intestinal parasites.

Strawberries

Early pharmacopoeias list strawberries as a remedy for constipation and skin complaints, including acne. They're naturally diuretic and mildly laxative. Unfortunately for some of us, these 'best of berries' can be a common cause of allergy, causing patchy skin rashes or hives. Some practitioners have suggested that the incidence of strawberry rash may have something to do with availability. In the shops for only a few short weeks each year, it's all too easy to overload the system by eating large quantities at one serving rather than just a few berries at a time. If you can't eat them, try smashing a few up in a blender with egg white and oatmeal to make a delicious face pack for oily skin. For those who can eat them, they're nothing if not nutritious. The revered naturopath and father of natural medicine, Dr Alfred Vogel, founder of the herbal medicine company Bioforce, was a great believer in the power of the strawberry plant. He recommended the fruit for its vitamin C content and as a blood purifier. An infusion of young strawberry leaves, he advocated, was a rich source of minerals, especially calcium.

FOLLOW THE FRUIT RULE

To obtain the maximum nutrient value from your fruit, follow the food-combining guidelines and enjoy it as a between-meal snack, an early morning juice or at the beginning of a meal – in other words, always on an empty stomach. And avoid the common practice of eating an apple or fruit salad as a dessert, especially not after a sandwich or any meal that contains starch. Piling the fruit – which requires a fast transit through the digestive system – on top of slow-moving protein or starch can mean that nothing will be broken down properly; fermentation and incomplete digestion will result, leading to bloating, flatulence, heartburn and abdominal discomfort.

With the exception of melon, which I would recommend is eaten entirely separately, all other fruits will mix happily with each other as long as there are no proteins or starches present. So enjoy a mixed fruit salad – but on its own.

Vegetables, Salad Foods and Sprouts

Artichokes

Globe artichokes are a valuable source of calcium, iron, vitamin C, thiamin, niacin and dietary fibre. They have powerful diuretic properties and are good for cleaning the liver and the kidneys which, in turn, helps the skin.

Asparagus

Another good internal cleanser, an excellent kidney tonic and a worthwhile source of vitamins C and E. Said to be good for all kinds of rheumatic and arthritic ailments. Fresh asparagus has such a short season, so make use of it when it is around, either steamed and served with a little melted butter or cold in salads with extra virgin olive oil. Asparagus is one of the few acid-forming vegetables (most are alkaline-forming), but it's nourishing none the less. And don't be alarmed if your urine smells slightly different on the day or day after you have eaten asparagus; its acid-forming nature alters the odour, but this is not believed to be detrimental in any way.

Avocado

Really a fruit, but used most often with salads and in savoury dishes, avocados are skin-savers in more ways than one. Easy to digest and rich in vitamins A, C, E, some B vitamins and potassium, they also contain monounsaturated oils (see page 29), now known to be beneficial in the war against the bad (LDL) cholesterol (see page 31). Good for ulcers and inflammation of the mucous membrane. Don't avoid avocados if you are trying to cut calories: half an avocado with an olive oil-and-cider vinegar dressing is a filling, nourishing and sustaining snack at only 200 calories. Avocados also make wonderful skin treatments and are used widely in cosmetic and skin-care products. For a soothing face pack, mash one-quarter of a fresh avocado with a dessertspoonful of plain bio-yoghurt. Spread the mixture evenly over the face and neck and leave in place for 15 minutes. Rinse away with tepid water. To make a great hair conditioner, mix and mash half an avocado with a teaspoon of dark liquid honey and two teaspoons of extra virgin olive oil.

Bamboo Shoots

Tender bamboo shoots can be eaten either raw or cooked in boiling water for about 10 minutes. They contain vitamins A and C, small amounts of some B vitamins, calcium and iron. A valuable skin food because of their detoxifying talents. Also reported to be beneficial for bowel disorders and high blood pressure.

Barley

Highly regarded as a nutritious food, barley has been used in the treatment of diarrhoea and ulcers, cystitis and fever. It is known to strengthen the hair and nails. It may also be valuable for asthmatics since it contains a substance, hordenine, which relieves bronchial spasm.

Beetroot

The blood-builder, a wonderful liver, kidney and bladder tonic and especially beneficial when juiced with apples, carrots and grapes. Raw beetroot is a rich source of iron, vitamin A, vitamin C and calcium and contains other valuable nutrients which are excellent for healthy skin, for strengthening blood vessels, fighting infection, for anaemia and heavy periods. Adding grapes to beetroot juice or beetroot salad is said to improve the absorption of nutrients. The strong colouring of urine and faeces caused by beetroot can be alarming but is, in fact, thought to be beneficial to the bowel, kidneys and bladder and not at all dangerous. Avoid pre-cooked beetroot, which usually contains preservatives.

Broccoli

Now known to contain a special anti-cancer chemical called sulphoraphane, broccoli is also a fund of vitamins and minerals including beta carotene, calcium, iron, folic acid and vitamins C and E. A wonderful vegetable for steaming or stir-frying, and delicious chopped raw into salads too.

Cabbage

Of all vegetables, this is probably the one most likely to bring back miserable memories of school dinners. But I'm not talking about the smelly, soggy sort here. Lightly steamed or shredded raw cabbage is a vital skin-saver. No need to eat it plain. Add a little sea salt, black pepper, extra virgin olive oil and/or organic balsamic vinegar. Cabbage water, although not a pleasant thought at breakfast time perhaps, is nevertheless a useful aid to digestion and a liver system- and blood-cleanser, making it an important skin food. Cabbage water is reputed to be good for the hair, nails, teeth, gums and bones. If the taste bothers you, try adding cooled cabbage water to a mixed vegetable juice or to organic carrot juice. Take care when cooking cabbage; its nutrients, particularly the valuable vitamin C content, are destroyed by prolonged cooking. Finely sliced raw cabbage is wonderful in coleslaw with grated apple, carrot, celery and onion.

Carrot

Carrots are high in fibre, vitamin C and beta carotene, the vegetable form of vitamin A. Great grated raw in salads and stir-fries, juiced, sliced for stews and casseroles or lightly steamed. The antioxidant properties of carrots are vital for healthy blood cells and healthy skin. Avoid the often unpleasant aftertaste of the mass-produced 'chemical' carrot by choosing organic carrots whenever they are available. (See page 67 for more info on organic foods.)

Celery and Celeriac

Celery is the stick-shaped stalk that grows out of celeriac, the celery root. Both are very nourishing and good in all kinds of hot and cold dishes, soups, stews, stir-fries and salads. The celeriac has more fibre than the celery stalks and is slightly richer in vitamin C. The green celery leaves are also good for you; shred them for salads or use for stocks and casseroles. Both celery and celeriac are good kidney-cleansers. All parts of the plant (and particularly the seeds) have long been recognized for their therapeutic value to arthritis sufferers.

In ancient texts, celery was prized as a blood-purifier and nerve tonic and is believed to be valuable for balancing blood pressure.

Chicory

Also known as Belgian endive or witloof. A super skin food with excellent cleansing properties. A tasty addition to salads and particularly enjoyable with apple and avocado. Curly endive is the green relative, a useful source of vitamin C, iron and beta carotene.

Cucumber

Cucumber extracts can be found in many cosmetic and skin-care products, particularly toners and cleansers, and it is easy to make your own preparations at home. Grate about a quarter of one whole cucumber and squeeze the juice into half a cupful of milk. Soak cotton pads with the mixture and use it as a cleanser. Or just whizz it up on its own for an effective skin toner. It suits all skin types. Cut slices of cucumber to pep up tired, gritty eyes and use cucumber skin to wipe over the face as an instant refresher.

Sea Vegetables

This general heading includes Chinese black moss, dulse, hijiki, kelp, kombu, mekabu, nori, plankton, wakame and other seaweeds. In some countries seaweed is available as a fresh vegetable food, but in others only in its dried form from health food stores and delicatessens. Prized by the ancient Greeks and Romans and the Chinese for their medicinal properties, seaweeds from non-toxic waters provide valuable minerals including calcium, chromium, cobalt, iron, iodine, manganese and zinc. It's not widely used in the UK, but is available worldwide. Nori, for example, has a world market of around 18 billion sheets (50 square centimetres or 8 square inches each) per year! Unfortunately, many seas are now so polluted that these once valuable vegetables may also be laced with nitrates and heavy metals such as cadmium, lead, strontium and mercury. Ask your health store about organic sources of seaweed for use in cooking.

Sprouted Seeds/Beans/Grains

One of the most nourishing food groups ever and wonderfully good for the skin. Try sprouting aduki beans, alfalfa, chick peas, fenugreek seeds, lentils, millet, mung beans, pumpkin seeds, sesame seeds or sunflower seeds. Fresh sprouts are an abundant source of nourishment – rich in enzymes, vitamin C, essential fatty acids, minerals, amino acids and natural sugars. They are also one of the cheapest foods around, making for a really tasty way of adding nutrition points without adding cost. During germination the concentration of nutrients increases many fold, providing the body with high-energy, low-calorie, nutrient-dense sustenance.

Preparing your own sprouts is simplicity itself. Specially designed kits are available from health food stores, but clean jam jars are just as easy to use and produce excellent results. Buy your seeds, beans and grains in small amounts and use them regularly. Check them over carefully and discard any damaged or broken ones. Rinse them thoroughly through a sieve, then fill each jar one-quarter full with your chosen beans, grains or seeds, topping up with filtered water. Use either a separate jar for each variety or mix them in the same jar if you prefer. Leave to soak overnight. In the morning, pour off the water, rinse them and top up with fresh water. Repeat the procedure two or three times each day (more in hot weather). Most sprouts will be ready in three or four days; some take longer. For more detailed information on sprouting, read Leslie Kenton's *Raw Energy*.

! **In the Know**
The darker green a vegetable is, the more vitamin C, beta carotene, iron and calcium it contains – up to six times as much as a paler counterpart. Dandelion greens, dark green cabbage and lettuce, turnip greens and kale are particularly nourishing skin foods. Choose dark-leaved lettuce, too.

Herbs

Burdock Root (*Arctium lappa*)

Prized for its medicinal value, burdock is often partnered with dandelion or artichoke in herbal treatments. It has natural antibiotic properties, is a great liver tonic and detoxifier, an energy-booster and restorative – a must in any detoxification programme – rich in iron, organic sulphur and B vitamins. Burdock has a cleansing effect upon the tissues and is recommended where mucus is a problem – such as in catarrh, sinusitis or mucus-laden stools – and for skin disorders, particularly boils, sores, poor wound-healing, dry skin and eczema. Burdock root is also available for use as a fresh vegetable (try Asian or Chinese food stores). Thin roots are the best; around 2¹/₂ centimetres (1 inch) in diameter. Scrub thoroughly and slice or grate for use in stir-fries or casseroles. Burdock has a mild, earthy flavour and a crunchy texture.

Dandelion (*Taraxacum officinale*)

For those who do not have access to fresh dandelion leaves or root, tablets and capsules are available from health food stores. Dandelion is a natural diuretic, one of the best kidney, liver and gall bladder tonics. Both the root and the leaves are excellent skin treatments, particularly where there is inflammation. Warts can be treated by applying the white sap directly to the affected areas. When treating skin disorders in my own patients, I have found dandelion and burdock to be two of the best remedies. Don't harvest dandelion leaves from the roadside – they could be contaminated with lead and other heavy metals. Always wash any collected leaves thoroughly before shredding and mixing with salads. The roots, dried, roasted or ground, make a caffeine-free coffee substitute. Most health food stores stock dandelion 'coffee'.

Garlic (*Allium satim*)

All members of the onion family, including leeks, shallots and chives, make great skin foods, but garlic is in the super league of face-savers. It has natural antiseptic, antibiotic, anti-viral and anti-fungal properties, is an excellent blood tonic, natural detoxifier, antioxidant and strengthener of immune function. Garlic has been used for centuries as a wound dressing and, in several trials, has demonstrated anti-tumour activity. In the *Medical Tribune* of August 1981, a report from China showed that those who did not eat garlic were a thousand times more prone to gastric cancer than those who ate large amounts. Onions and garlic taken throughout the winter months do seem to help ward off colds and other infections. Parsley, mint and orange, lemon or grapefruit peelings help to eliminate the odour of garlic from the breath. So does a glass of good red wine!

Although still of value, fresh garlic will lose a considerable amount of its therapeutic activity once cooked, so if you are unable to tolerate raw garlic, an alternative option may be to take it as a supplement. If you use garlic tablets or capsules, always swallow them half-way through a meal, rather than at the beginning or the end. This seems to help absorption, reduce any risk of indigestion and reduce the impact of any odour. Some brands of deodorized garlic don't seem to have the same beneficial effects as fresh, raw or aged garlic.

Tip: If you use fresh garlic in your juicing machine, the odour may cling and taint other juices. Overcome the problem by washing the machine parts in a solution of biodegradable cleaning fluid or sterilizing fluid which removes the smell of fish, onions and any other strong odours from hands, work surfaces, cooking utensils, etc.

Mint (*Mentha* x *piperita*)

Add flavour to stews, soups, salads and vegetables with chopped mint leaves. Or infuse whole leaves to make a stimulating tea (reputed to be helpful for arthritis) or to use as a refreshing mouth wash or hair rinse. Also of value as an air freshener and insect repellent.

Nettle (*Urtica dioica*)

The common nettle has astringent, diuretic, tonic, antirheumatic, circulatory stimulant and blood-purifying properties – all beneficial in the treatment of skin problems. Young nettle shoots are rich in vitamin C, beta carotene and mineral salts. Cook young nettle leaves like spinach (once cooked, they have no sting), make a tisane (tea) or use as a cleansing hair rinse – good for dandruff – and face tonic. But do take care to wear protective gloves if you decide to gather fresh leaves.

Parsley (*Petroselinum crispum*)

The green curly leaves of parsley are a rich source of vitamin C, beta carotene, potassium, calcium and important trace elements boron, manganese, molybdenum and zinc. A great herbal helper for the skin, parsley is delicious in both salads and cooked dishes. The juice of fresh parsley root helps in the healing of wounds and reduces swelling. Chew fresh parsley to remove garlic odour from the breath. Mix fresh parsley sprigs with your vegetable juices.

> **In the Know**
>
> Herbal Elixir from the Green People Company contains 12 nutritious organic plant juices including celery, dandelion, nettle, carrot, garlic and artichoke. Believed to help the inner cleansing process and boost the immune system, it is a worthwhile tonic if your energy is flagging or you're feeling sluggish. Add a teaspoon of Elixir to your daily juice.

Other Superskin Foods

Fish

All kinds of fish are good for you, but the oily ones such as mackerel, salmon, sardines and trout are particularly rich in special fatty substances called eicosapentaenoic acid (EPA) and docosahexaenoic acid (DHA), essential for healthy blood, cells and skin. Fish oil, available in capsules, is showing promise as a treatment both for psoriasis and high blood pressure and can be helpful as a general treatment for dry skin conditions.

Look out for quality fish oil supplements that detail the EPA and DHA content on the label. It's worth knowing that, if you eat oily fish twice a week, then you shouldn't need to take capsules as well.

NUTRITIONAL-GRADE LINSEED OIL

If you are allergic to – or simply don't eat – fish, then linseed oil is a valuable vegetarian alternative with similar nutritional properties. A truly superb skin food, it's available from good health stores and from the supplement supplier Biocare in capsule form and as a liquid from Savant Health (*see Resources chapter*).

Important note: The shelf-life of unadulterated cold-pressed linseed oil is short, so take care to store it in a cool, dark place. Buy it in small quantities and use up well before the 'sell by' date.

Oats

A wonderful supplier of calcium, iron, magnesium, potassium, silicon, vitamin E, B vitamins, essential fatty acids, protein and soluble dietary fibre. Apart from porridge, enjoy oat-based muesli, oat cakes and oat biscuits. Oats make a good gentle exfoliator; combine a dessertspoon of oatmeal with a teaspoon of honey and a few drops of jojoba or almond oil and massage it all into the face and neck. Do it over the washbasin or in the bath. Leave for 5 minutes, then rinse. For a terrific face-pack for dry, flaky or cracked skin, mix a handful with yoghurt and avocado. Messy but brilliant. To soothe eczema, fill a muslin bag or a clean kneehigh stocking (popsock) with organic oatmeal and squidge it around in the bath water while you soak.

Extra Virgin Olive Oil

One of life's most important skin-savers; adding nutritious cold-pressed oils to the diet is one of the best ways to improve skin texture and moisturize from within. Rich in monounsaturated oils, now known to be extremely beneficial for healthy blood, healthy skin and for all kinds of gall bladder and liver ailments, extra virgin olive oil is guaranteed by law to be untreated by chemicals. Studies show olive oil to be helpful in balancing both blood cholesterol and blood glucose. It is highly rated as a nerve tonic, tissue-strengthener and constipation remedy. Include a tablespoon per day in salad dressings or for stir-frying, even if you are following a low-fat diet. Use it externally for sunburn, minor skin eruptions and massage. Olive oil is also useful for scalp massage and as a general hair treatment. Always make sure you buy 'Extra Virgin', 'Virgin' or 'First Pressing' cold-pressed olive oil. And choose organic oil wherever possible. Labels which simply say 'Pure' are not of the same high grade.

Wholegrain Rice

Brown rice provides B vitamins, calcium, magnesium, iron, zinc and gentle dietary fibre. It is easily digested and has amazing absorptive qualities for it soaks up toxins from the gut and transports them from the body. To maintain a healthy skin, detoxification and efficient elimination of wastes is vital. Brown rice is one of the best sources of skin-clearing fibre. Eat plenty of other wholegrains too; there's lots of variety available, such as bulgur, couscous, millet, oat bran, brown pasta, quinoa and rye.

Yoghurt

One of those skin foods which is just as good for the inside of the body as it is for the outside skin, yoghurt provides protein, calcium, magnesium, potassium, zinc, thiamin, riboflavin and vitamin A (although there is less vitamin A in the low-fat varieties). Always choose plain yoghurts that are 'live' or 'bio' and check for *Lactobacillus acidophilus* or other healthy bacteria on the label. I have always found sheep's milk and goat's milk yoghurt more suited to my skin than cow's milk products.

Include a small tub of good-quality sheep's or goat's yoghurt once or twice a week. They're now widely available in health stores and supermarkets as an alternative to cow's milk. If you've been devoted to the regular low-fat yoghurts, check the labels for additives, stabilizers and emulsifiers, often added to replace the fat content. It could be healthier to eat a little less of the unadulterated full-fat version than more additives. On the outside, yoghurt is a nourishing face pack. The lactic acid content acts like a natural exfoliator; in a similar way to the alpha hydroxy acids (AHAs) which turn up in skin care products but without the danger of allergic reactions which have been associated with AHAs. Plain yoghurt also makes a soothing douche or cream application for vaginal thrush. For more information on yoghurt and milk, see pages 50 and 62 and my books *The Food Combining Diet* (Thorsons) or *The Complete Book of Food Combining* (Piatkus).

Honey

This delectable sweetener has been part of the human diet since time immemorial, first as wild honey and then 'cultivated' in man-made hives; it was used by the ancient Greeks and Romans and recommended by Hippocrates. The subject of wealthy anecdotal evidence, honey certainly would seem to have some medicinal properties. Mixed with cider vinegar, it makes a soothing cough and sore throat remedy. Some types of honey are said to be helpful for easing the pain of arthritis. A report in the *British Journal of Surgery* (1991; 78: 497–8) showed honey to be beneficial in the treatment of superficial burns, helping wounds to heal faster than conventional treatments. It can also be a useful 'stepping stone' for people trying to cut down on sugar. The sugar in honey is called *levulose* (related to the fruit sugar, fructose) and, because much of it can be absorbed into the liver without the use of insulin, puts less of a strain on the pancreas. Ordinary sugar (sucrose) needs insulin before it can be broken down and utilized. Contrary to common belief, brown sugar is no more nutritious than white. In addition, sucrose is itself nutritionally dead and has a nasty habit of using up or destroying other nutrients in the body. Good-quality honey, on the other hand, especially the darker coloured varieties, contains trace amounts of vitamins and minerals.

When choosing honey, read the labels with care. Many will use the words 'produce of more than one country' or 'blended', indicating that several honeys have been heated to mix them together. Overheating can destroy nutrients, so it's best to choose single-source honey from a reputable supplier. It's worth bearing in mind that although organic honey, free from pesticide sprays, is likely to be a better option, the word 'organic' isn't going to mean much if the honey concerned has been heat-treated. A good guide is price: cheaper honey is nearly always blended. Some inferior brands will also lack nutrients if the bees' diet has been supplemented with sugar solution. Honey still on the comb is usually a good option. If you are in doubt about where to buy your honey, check out your local health food store. Always choose cold-pressed honey and buy the best that you can afford. My favourite honey, called Manuka, comes from the flowers of the same New Zealand plant that produces Manuka essential oil. Not only is it nutritious but it has natural anti-bacterial properties too. Page 229 has stockist details.

Molasses

Apart from honey, the only other sugar which is not 'pure, white and deadly' is molasses. This unrefined extraction from the sugar cane contains traces of vitamins and some important minerals – calcium, magnesium, iron, potassium, silicon and sulphur. Another 'old' arthritis remedy, molasses is also rich in phosphoric acid, an essential cell builder which was once given to children to help improve growth and cure anaemia. A useful – and nutritious – alternative sweetener.

Nuts

These concentrated foods are often dismissed by slimmers as fattening but, although some nuts can be high in calories, they have high energy value too and are nutrient-dense. They provide valuable dietary fibre, monounsaturated and polyunsaturated oils (see page 29), worthwhile levels of protein and important minerals such as calcium, magnesium, iron and zinc. Nuts best for skin are unblanched almonds, brazils, pine nuts and macadamias. Nuts are an extremely concentrated food and so should be consumed in moderation only. The oils they contain are prone to rancidity, so proper storage is essential. Top-quality nuts will be unbroken (preferably still in their shells) and sold in sealed bags with a clearly marked 'use by' date. Keep them in a cool dark cupboard and do not expose them to daylight or hot kitchens. If flaked nuts are required for a particular dish or recipe, break them up in a coffee grinder or processor as you need them.

Peanuts are actually members of the pulse family and can cause allergic reactions in some people. Unless absolutely fresh, they can carry aflatoxins (present in a fungus often invisible to the naked eye) which are potentially carcinogenic. Salted, roasted nuts are a delicious indulgence, but are not good skin foods – not just because of the salt content but because the structure of the oils they contain may have been altered in the roasting process.

Seeds

Like nuts, seeds are a concentrated food source rich in unsaturated oils (see page 31) – excellent for the skin. Correct storage is, once again, vital so buy them in small amounts and keep them in a screw-top jar in the refrigerator. Don't choose seeds (or nuts) from serve-yourself hoppers – they will have been exposed to heat, light and air which hastens degeneration. Sunflower seeds, pumpkin seeds, linseeds, almonds, walnuts, brazils, macadamia nuts and hazelnuts all contain essential fatty acids and so make terrific skin foods. Caraway, celery, dill, fennel, fenugreek, poppy and sesame seeds are also excellent. Avoid roasted ones; the oils they contain are likely to have been damaged.

⸙ Skin Scoundrels

The foods listed here are, in my view, unlikely to help you towards healthy skin. Enjoy the occasional indulgence without feeling guilty, but avoid excesses. Too many of the 'bad guy' foods will simply undo all your good work.

☒ **All beef and beef products – apart from occasional meals of organically reared beef**

☒ All pork and pork products – including ham, pig's liver, pork pies, sausages and bacon; if you like meat, enjoy lean lamb instead

☒ Fatty lamb

☒ Preserved, smoked meats or smoked fish

☒ Processed, coloured or smoked cheeses

☒ Foods that contain long lists of E numbers and chemical-sounding names

☒ Fatty and fried foods – especially take-aways

☒ Refined sugar in all its forms – chocolate, sweets, ice cream, cakes, biscuits, sweet pastries, doughnuts, jam, etc.

☒ Any food which is burned, browned, seared or barbecued

☒ Highly spiced foods

☒ Foods with added salt and salty snacks

☒ White bread and any foods containing refined flour

☒ Wheat bran and wheat-based breakfast cereals

☒ Dried milks, dried eggs, powdered soups and coffee creamers

☒ Highly refined or processed foods and 'ready' meals

☒ Canned foods (exceptions: sardines, tuna and salmon, which are good sources of fish oil and calcium, and fruit in natural juice, a useful emergency standby)

☒ Polyunsaturated margarines if they contain hydrogenated oils; and please don't cook with polyunsaturates of any kind (see page 31)

☒ Cow's milk and cow's milk cheeses (see page 50)

☒ Yeast and yeasty foods

☒ Watch out for low-fat cheeses, spreads and yoghurts – emulsifiers, stabilizers, artificial flavours and colours are often used to replace the fat

☒ Excessive amounts of coffee, tea, cola, alcohol and squashes; they aggravate dehydration and increase the risk of tiny red surface veins

☒ Foods that fight (i.e. proteins mixed with starches – see page 82) or any food combined with fruit

Note: Foods containing sugar or yeast are also to be avoided if you suffer from *candidiasis,* a condition where an overgrowth of the yeast *Candida albicans* can produce a multitude of physical symptoms, notably the development or aggravation of skin problems. Following an anti-Candida diet can be very beneficial but it should be done under expert supervision, so if you think you may have this condition do consult a naturopath or dermatologist who specializes in its treatment.

For more information on *Candida albicans* and the treatment of candidiasis, read *The Practical Guide to Candida* by Jane McWhirter (Green Library).

✱ Fat Facts

I'm fat but I'm thin inside. Has it ever struck you that there's a thin man inside every fat man, just as they say there's a statue inside every block of stone.

GEORGE ORWELL (ERIC ARTHUR BLAIR, 1903–50), *COMING UP FOR AIR*

Why Certain Fats and Oils Are Vital for Healthy Skin

I cover the subject of fats and oils in some detail because getting the balance right is absolutely crucial for skin health. Let's face it, whether it's on your hips or in your chips, fat has become an obsession. But the all-consuming media attention given to this villain of the diet-piece has done little to curtail the nation's corpulence or to correct its health problems.

And now a new 'illness' may be creeping upon us as a result of such extreme abstinence. Fat neurosis has brought with it 'Fat Deficiency Disorders', something which I've found frequently in new patients who come to my nutrition practice: a real fear of eating anything that contains or resembles fat for fear of becoming fat or of contracting heart disease or high cholesterol.

A typical scenario is the woman who, approaching the menopause, begins to put on a bit of extra weight (often nothing more than a natural consequence of ageing and which has the benefit of providing added protection against osteoporosis, the dreaded 'brittle bone disease'). In her paranoid panic over those few additional pounds, she goes on to a 'low-fat diet' which is really a 'no-fat' diet. Common sense for good health, you might say. In moderation, certainly reducing fat intake is believed to help lessen the risk of degenerative disease and can help to reduce weight – but taking these recommendations to extremes may cause more problems than it solves and can be particularly damaging to skin health.

Why?

Don't Take Low-fat Dieting Too Far

By cutting down too far on certain types of fat, especially those unrefined liquid oils, we run the risk of becoming deficient in some very special substances called essential fatty acids. EFAs are needed by all cells in the body and are the most plentiful constituent in the membrane – or fabric – that surrounds each and every cell. Fundamental and indispensable skin nutrients, EFAs help to reduce water loss from the cells, protecting the lipidic barrier between each layer of skin and preventing evaporation. They also help to build collagen and elastin fibres so, without EFAs, the plumpness and firmness of the skin is diminished, encouraging sagging, drooping and wrinkling!

EFAs play an important part in a healthy nervous system too, feeding the nerve endings and sensory receptors in the skin.

Unrefined food oils are also a rich source of fatty vitamins (A, D and E) and lecithin, which acts to prevent the build-up of undesirable blocking fats, thereby reducing the risk of infection associated with oily skin, acne, spots and blemishes. Lecithin is also a very effective lubricant for dry skin.

Diets which go to fat-reducing extremes no longer contain sufficient of these vital nutrients and a list of unpleasant symptoms begin to manifest. Most common are:

※ Dry, flaky skin
※ Brittle nails
※ Lifeless hair
※ Joint pain and stiffness
※ Extreme coldness of the hands and feet
※ Vaginal dryness
※ Persistent viral infections
※ Difficult periods
※ Pre-menstrual syndrome
※ Breast pain
※ Loss of skin texture and premature wrinkles.

These are signs that the cells may not be receiving the protection they need. More severe deficiencies could lead to inflammatory conditions such as arthritis, damage to the immune system and, believe it or not, heart disease. If any of the above symptoms apply to you and have become worse since you cut your fat intake, make sure that you haven't cut back too far.

There is no getting away from the fact that fat is a mandatory body nutrient. Its Nemesis lies not so much in its use but in its mis-use, either inside the body or before it is consumed. Where the diet contains the wrong kinds of fats and oils in large amounts, trouble may brew. On the other hand, the right kinds in sensible quantities are absolutely, positively and definitely necessary for good health. Good skin is an impossible achievement without them and understanding the difference between good and bad fats and oils is essential in the quest for that perfect complexion.

What Goes Wrong?

It's not fat which causes disease, but what happens to it when it is attacked by oxygen, i.e. oxidized – like perished rubber, rusty cans and cars, or apples which go brown. Oxygen is, of course, the breath of life but, in certain circumstances, it can also act as a poison. When fats, oils and fatty foods oxidize, they 'go off' and become rancid. And fats inside the body can be attacked in a similar way, turning our natural body fats (or lipids) rancid; a process called lipid peroxidation.

Free Radical Felons

Some fats degrade more readily than others, but all fats will deteriorate rapidly given 'favourable' conditions. The result is an over-production of highly active chemical compounds called free radicals, unstable substances produced as a direct result of oxygen assault.

In a healthy body, the free radicals produced a result of normal metabolic processes are kept in check and even offer some health benefits – albeit limited. When out of control, however, free radicals behave like bad-tempered bachelors out to steal someone else's partner.

What Are the Dangers?

Within the body, oxygen atoms could be considered a partnership, living together as a 'twosome'. The strength of their 'marriage' depends upon the protection supplied by the body's Argus-eyed free radical scavengers. When supplies are short, when the diet contains an overdose of undesirable fats or when the body is exposed excessively to pollution, radiation, infection, stress, smoking, etc., the security screen is less effective, allowing unruly unwed free radicals to break up the relationship.

But this spouse-swapping doesn't affect just one couple. As the fanatical free radicals whizz around the body in a desperate search for a partner to join up with, they create a roller-coaster effect which produces new free radicals, all out to make more mischief. The resulting havoc damages cells, causing tissues to become cross-linked (a wrinkle is the result of cross-linkage), suppressing the manufacture of new healthy cells, reducing the body's ability to fight infection and to repair damage – in other words, encouraging premature ageing and degenerative disease.

Each cell in the body is governed by its own 'clock', programmed to tick for a certain length of time before running down and finally switching off. While ageing and degeneration are inevitable, there are ways of shielding the system against this devastating onslaught and slowing its decline. One of those ways is to support the system with super-nutritious, antioxidant-rich food.

The Antioxidant Armoury

The body has a variety of protective and scavenging mechanisms stock-piled against free-radical attack. Antioxidants are the vitamins, minerals and enzymes which protect cells from oxidation (degeneration). Important antioxidant enzymes are supported by antioxidant nutrients from the diet and together they guard the cellular structure. Mother Nature also adds antioxidants (such as vitamins A, C and E, beta carotene and minerals selenium and zinc) to foods which contain susceptible fats and oils – for example, nuts, seeds and vegetables.

Trouble is, this armour is not always enough. Damaging sunlight, heat, air (oxygen, again) and radiation can speed up the oxidation process – one of the reasons why fats and oils which are reheated, overheated or left unrefrigerated in hot kitchens turn rancid so easily.

Once inside the body, degeneration can continue and will only be contained and controlled if the person's diet provides them with the antioxidant protection they need. Research shows that increasing your intake of antioxidant nutrients guards against damaging oxidation and helps to mop up free radicals, thereby slowing down the rate at which cells age and die. (For more information concerning antioxidants, vitamins and minerals, see Chapter 2.)

Evidence is emerging that these protectors may be a more significant and positive factor in the fight against ageing and disease than worrying unnecessarily over the actual levels of dietary fat.

We Need Fat

Fat gives structure, substance, palatability and flavour to food. Take it out of yoghurts, spreads, ice cream, cheeses or mayonnaise and they would turn into a nasty watery squidgy mess of nothing very appetizing. That's why manufacturers of low-fat foods so often add 'supports' such as stabilizers, binders, fillers, bulking agents, flavourings and preservatives to glue the fat-free remnants back together. Taking away the fat could also mean losing out on fat-soluble nutrients such as vitamins A and E, as well as those all-important EFAs that I was talking about earlier.

So What About Those Low-fat Foods?

In the pursuit of fat-reduction, many people rely on processed products such as low-fat cheeses, low-fat yoghurts and reduced-calorie mayonnaise and fromage frais. While the official advice is that these foods are perfectly healthy, I am concerned that we may be storing up further problems for the future by swapping unadulterated fat for additives and hydrogenated oils.

Why Do We Like Fat So Much?

Fat fills us up and takes longer to digest than other foods; that's why, if we eat a meal with a high fat content, we feel full for longer. Hence the comfort gained from chips, crisps, cakes, pastries, doughnuts, fry-ups, etc.

What Do Saturated, Monounsaturated and Polyunsaturated Really Mean?

Fat is made up of molecules of fatty acids combined with a substance called glycerol. Each molecule is a chain-like structure of carbon atoms to which hydrogen atoms are attached. It is the shape of each structure that determines whether the fat is saturated, monounsaturated or polyunsaturated.

Sources of:

Saturates	Monounsaturates	Polyunsaturates
Dripping	Almond	Corn (Maize)
Suet	Avocado	Fish oil
Lard	Cashew	Grapeseed
Hard margarine	Hazelnut	Linseed
Cream	Macadamia	Pumpkin seed
Cheese	Olive	Rapeseed
Milk	Pecan	Safflower
Fatty meats	Pistachio	Sesame*
Coconut		Sunflower
Butter		Walnut

*   *Brazil nuts, pine nuts, sesame seeds (and the oils produced from them) contain approximately equal amounts of monounsaturated and polyunsaturated oils and should therefore be treated with the respect afforded to all other polyunsaturates; in other words, avoid heating them. While some authorities state that sesame oil is suitable for cooking because of its monounsaturate content, the poly-unsaturates it contains are still susceptible to damage. I would therefore strongly recommend that sesame oil and seeds be kept for cold uses only.*

Sorting the Good from the Not So Good

Saturates

Saturates are those fats that tend to be solid at room temperature, like butter. Full-fat milk, cheese, cream and fatty meats are rich in saturates, the kind of fat we are usually advised to cut down on. Note, however, that there have never been any recommendations that we should give up satu-rated fats entirely; the body could not function properly without them. The problems lie in excess intake. Saturates can clog the arteries and slow the passage of blood and nutrients through the system. They can also overwork the lymph system (part of the body's detoxifying defences) and make it difficult for the internal 'refuse collectors' to take out the garbage. The routes of elimination become overburdened with the consequent build-up of 'junk' and the skin tries to take over some of the work. Result? Clogged pores, excess oil, pale and pasty complexion, blemishes, acne, body odour, lethargy.

Perhaps the best advice is this: be sensible about saturates. Use them and enjoy them, but in moderation only. We could all do with cutting down just a little, but there's no need to give up butter entirely.

Monounsaturates

These are found in avocado pear and olive oil and many of the nuts like macadamia and almond. Research shows that monounsaturated oils can be helpful in balancing blood glucose (good for people with diabetes or hypoglycaemia alike) and reducing the less desirable low-density lipoprotein (LDL) cholesterol without disturbing the levels of the beneficial high-density lipoprotein (HDL) cholesterol. Check the table on page 30 to find the most abundant sources of monounsaturates.

Official guidelines now recommend that these important oils should provide 12 per cent of total dietary energy. Monounsaturates also make wonderful skin, hair and nail conditioners, which you'll find out more about in Part Three.

Polyunsaturates

These have, for several years, been promoted as the healthy alternative to saturates and as synonymous with lowering cholesterol. Following this advice, many people dutifully dismissed their butter and jumped earnestly on to the polyunsaturated bandwagon. Unfortunately, as with so many things dietary, that counsel is now being challenged and re-examined. One of the problems is that, while helping to cut levels of the LDL cholesterol, polyunsaturated fatty acids (PUFAs) also reduce HDL (the cholesterol we would rather hang on to), throwing the ratio out of balance. The most important thing to know is that the quality of PUFAs in tubs of spread is probably not going to be as good as natural polyunsaturates from unprocessed sources.

The simplest way to picture a polyunsaturated oil is as a supple and pliable chain of double links with kinks in them. It's the bendy nature of the structure which makes the oil fluid. Truly healthy 'polys' are those found in nut, seed and vegetable foods and in fish. The natural state of the oil extracted from these foods is liquid, not solid. If the oil is pressed out of, say, a pumpkin seed or an olive without the use of heat or chemical solvents, it remains a rich source of those very important skin nutrients that we talked about on page 25, essential fatty acids.

The not-so-good news is that the vast majority of mass-produced liquid oils which we find on the shelves of our food stores (sunflower, corn, grapeseed, etc.) are heated and processed using solvents – which not only alter their structure but can reduce their nutritional value. Some experts believe that the chemical changes that take place during processing can even be dangerous to the human body.

HYDROGENATION

I'll describe the process to you and then leave you to make up your own mind. Most spreads are made using a process called hydrogenation (look on your margarine label for the words 'hydrogenated vegetable oil'). This involves heating the liquid oil under high pressure for several hours, mixing in some hydrogen gas and adding chemical solvents, deodorizers and bleaching agents. The process alters the chemical structure by filling up the spaces in those flexible links so that the chain becomes straight and solid, having the effect of changing some of the polyunsaturates into saturates. Hydrogenation also removes large amounts of vitamin E, beta carotene and lecithin and destroys a considerable number of the beneficial EFAs, turning them into potentially unhealthy trans fatty acids or TFAs. Some research suggests that TFAs could be responsible for raised cholesterol, increased cell damage and lowered immunity. Doesn't sound too good a deal, does it?

If you cook using polyunsaturated oils, you could be damaging them in a similar way, especially if the oil is reheated. Just keep in mind that mass-produced oils which state 'suitable for frying' have more to with the fact that the oil is less likely to spit when heated than whether or not it is truly safe to use.

Note: Since there is unlikely to be smoke without fire, it may, perhaps, be premature to treat hydrogenated oils as safe until proven otherwise. My nutritionist's instincts incline me to the more guarded approach that we should avoid them until their benefits/hazards have been evaluated objectively and independently by researchers who can declare no vested interests in the food industry or its sales.

POLYUNSATURATES FALL INTO TWO GROUPS

Real polyunsaturates are not spreading fats, but oils found mainly in vegetables, nuts, seeds and oily fish. Corn, grapeseed, safflower and sunflower are the most familiar of the polyunsaturated oils found on our grocery or supermarket shelves. Once extracted from their host plant, real polys remain naturally liquid at room temperature. If undamaged by processing and carefully stored, they are rich in essential fatty acids and of great value to the diet. The body cannot produce its own polyunsaturated fatty acids and it is imperative that these vital nutrients are provided from the food we eat.

To Get the Most from Your Fats and Oils, Follow These Simple Rules:

❋ Choose the best quality oils you can find. Price is a reliable guide, since the more expensive oils are nearly always more nutritious. Look for the words 'cold pressed' on the label, indicating that the oil has not been damaged by overprocessing or the use of solvents. Health food stores generally have a better selection than most supermarkets.

❋ Buy in small quantities and use up well before the recommended date.

❋ Never, never, never use polyunsaturates of any kind for anything that requires heating or cooking. The increase in temperature encourages the formation of lipid peroxides, dangerous and potentially carcinogenic substances. So, keep them for salad dressings and mayonnaise only. Chips cooked in polyunsaturated oil are not healthier than those cooked in animal fat!

❋ Don't leave oils standing in a hot kitchen or in daylight, two of the speediest ways to turn them rancid. Store them in a cool, dark cupboard or, better still, in the refrigerator. I believe that manufacturers should be encouraged to use dark glass bottles instead of clear glass or plastic.

❋ Always replace the cap securely.

❋ If you use polyunsaturated spreads, check the label and avoid those that are made using hydrogenated vegetable oils. Choose non-hydrogenated spreads which have been made without heat treatment or solvents.

In the Know

The health-giving structure of polyunsaturates is altered, detrimentally, if they are over-processed, heated, subjected to light, air, radiation or environmental pollution, stripped of their natural antioxidant protectors – such as vitamin E – or hydrogenated.

Here's How to Cut Fat Intake But Still Enjoy Real Food!

1 Eat more fresh fish and free-range poultry.
2 Cut down on red meat, particularly beefburgers, sausages, bacon, pork pies and pasties.
3 Be sensible about sticky buns, cakes, biscuits, chocolate, ice cream and crisps. Enjoy them only as very occasional treats.

4   Stir-fry, grill, poach, bake or casserole your food. Never deep-fry anything.

5   Use extra virgin olive oil (instead of polyunsaturates) for cooking. It's more stable when heated and less prone to rancidity (although careful storage guidelines still apply).

6   For spreading, avoid margarines that are made with hydrogenated vegetable oils (check the labels) and use either small amounts of butter or non-hydrogenated spreads – available from health food stores.

7   Avoid low-fat foods of the processed variety, especially if they contain lots of artificial additives and chemical-sounding names.

8   If you can't decide between low-fat cheeses, yoghurts or mayonnaise which contain lots of artificial additives and full-fat alternatives which don't, then I would say go for the latter but eat half the amount.

9   Try to avoid cow's milk altogether. Instead, use soya milk for cooking and for milky drinks. On cereals, try rice milk or oat milk. My great indulgence is an absolutely delicious hot chocolate which I make with Green & Black's Organic Chocolate Powder and Provamel Organic Soya Milk. Not sickly sweet, but nourishing and refreshing. All these products are readily available from larger supermarkets and most health stores.

chapter 2

Vital Skin Nutrients

A good kitchen is a good Apothecary's shop.
WILLIAM BULLEIN (D. 1576), *THE BULWARK AGAINST ALL SICKNESS*

A keen gardener may spend hours digging, weeding and hoeing the beds and borders in order to produce a beautifully manicured appearance. But if the nutrients in the soil are lacking or are not replaced, then the plants growing there will eventually suffer. Skin is a lot like that. Take it for granted, ignore its needs, don't feed it properly – and it will suffer. And in the same way that plants take most of their nourishment from below the ground, skin health depends on nutrients from inside the body. If the body is poorly nourished and lacking in the vitamins, minerals, amino-acids, enzymes and hormones that all act synergistically to renew healthy cells, the skin can't be fed either. So let's look at what these vital nutrients can do to help your skin.

First up, it can be really helpful to know where to find those all-important skin nutrients we hear so much about – *antioxidants*, as well as some of the other vitamins and minerals that are essential to healthy skin.

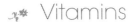 Vitamins

Vitamin A

Vitamin A is an essential skin nutrient and is found in the diet in two basic forms:

1   *Beta carotene* is an important anti-ageing nutrient found in carotenoid foods; for example, cantaloupe melons, apricots, pumpkins, carrots, swedes, turnips, parsley, endive, squash, sweet potatoes, plankton and dark green leafy vegetables. In fact, most orange, yellow and dark green produce contains beta carotene. It's also what's known as 'a precursor of vitamin A'; in other words, in ideal conditions the body will convert beta carotene into vitamin A in the small intestine and liver. Beta carotene also has a separate role as an antioxidant, protecting cells from damage.

> In the Know
> Carotene was first discovered and named in 1919 when a yellow/orange pigment was extracted from carrots. It is beta carotene that gives organic and free-range egg yolks their natural orange colour, supplied to the hens by the vegetable foods in their feed. Many battery-raised eggs contain artificial colouring in their yolks.

2   *Retinol* is the name given to the vitamin A available from animal foods such as lamb's liver, oily fish, fish oil supplements, eggs and cheese. This vitamin is fat soluble and is stored by the body (unlike water-soluble vitamins such as the B complex which get washed out of the system every day). Because excesses of vitamin A can be toxic, nutritionists and doctors usually advise caution. However, in reality, too much from the diet alone would be difficult to achieve and there is no evidence that the small amounts of vitamin A in multivitamin supplements are anything other than

beneficial. It's worth knowing that deficiencies are as dangerous as excesses. Vitamin A is essential to a strong immune system and also to a healthy pregnancy. Studies show its importance in the prevention and treatment of dangerous childhood illnesses such as measles. From your skin's point of view, a lack of vitamin A can lead to slow wound-healing and to the damage of cell membranes. If new cells die off before they have a chance to reach the surface, this can block pores and prevent lubrication of the skin.

(Retinol is not to be confused with the vitamin A-based drug Retin A.)

Both kinds of vitamin A are widely available from food and yet borderline deficiencies are more common than you might think.

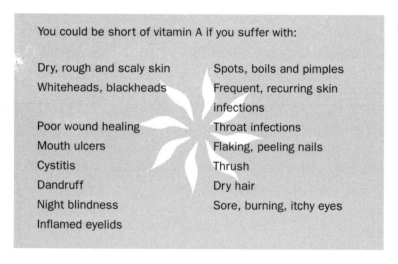

You could be short of vitamin A if you suffer with:

Dry, rough and scaly skin

Whiteheads, blackheads

Poor wound healing

Mouth ulcers

Cystitis

Dandruff

Night blindness

Inflamed eyelids

Spots, boils and pimples

Frequent, recurring skin infections

Throat infections

Flaking, peeling nails

Thrush

Dry hair

Sore, burning, itchy eyes

Vitamin A enhances the activity of essential fatty acids, particularly gamma linolenic acid (GLA); it works closely with zinc to support immune function and helps to transport other life-sustaining nutrients to the cells. A good deal of scientific research has shown vitamin A to be linked to reducing the risk of cancer; long-term studies continue, with promising results.

Where to Find Beta Carotene

Apricots

Asparagus

Broccoli

Cantaloupe melon

Carrots

Cashew nuts

Cauliflower greens

Cheese

Nectarines

Parsley

Peaches

Bell peppers

Pumpkin

Spinach

Spring greens

Sweet potatoes

Turnip tops

Watercress

Where to Find Vitamin A

Butter

Cheese

Cod liver oil

Free-range eggs

Halibut liver oil

Lamb's liver

Oily fish

The B Complex Group

Includes:

Thiamin (B_1)

Riboflavin (B_2)

Nicotinic Acid – sometimes also called Niacin (B_3)

Pantothenic Acid (B_5)

Pyridoxine (B_6)

Folic Acid (B_9)

Cobalamin (B_{12})

Biotin (also known as vitamin H)

Choline and inositol are also members of the B group, but are not strictly vitamins since they can be manufactured within the body. Para-aminobenzoic acid (PABA) is also part of this group, but should be regarded as a B factor, not a true vitamin.

Vitamin B deficiency symptoms include:

Pale skin	Generally poor skin condition
Cracks, splits or sores around the nose and mouth	Sore, itchy eyes
Pre-menstrual syndrome	Irregular, heavy or painful periods
Extreme fatigue	Lack of energy
Twitchy, restless limbs	Tingling or 'burning' in the legs or arms
Difficulty with memory	A tendency to drop or bump into things
Nervous disorders	Panic attacks
Dry, lacklustre hair	Brittle nails

In the Know
Three B vitamins, namely B_6, B_{12} and folic acid, have been found to be especially important in preventing and reducing high levels of a rogue amino acid, called homocysteine, which increases the risk of heart disease.

B vitamins are needed for the repair and rebuilding of tissue, for feeding the endocrine and nervous systems and for energy production. If you're under prolonged negative stress, feel generally run down, unusually irritable or anxious, or are having difficulty sleeping, consider B complex.

Aim, always, to get as much nourishment as possible from your diet, but bear in mind that food processing, freezing, crop sprays, the contraceptive pill, cigarette smoke and diets high in sugar can all reduce the levels of B vitamins in the food supply. Most good-quality multi-formulas or B complexes will provide 25–50 mg of each B vitamin. Two good ones that I like very much are Biocare's Enzyme-Activated B Complex and Naturetime Executive B from Blackmores.

Where to Find the B Vitamins

Apricots	Oats
Avocado pears	Oily fish
Bananas	Peas and beans
Brown rice	Potatoes
Carrots	Pumpkins
Free-range chicken	Root and green vegetables
Free-range eggs	Rye flour
Dried fruits	Salad produce
All kinds of grains	Soya flour
Melons	Spirulina
Nuts	Yoghurt

Buzz Word

Riboflavin – also known as vitamin B_2 – has a natural orange colouring. That's why your urine appears darker orange when you begin to take B complex or multivitamins. Don't worry, this vitamin is very good for you and its colour is completely harmless.

Vitamin C

Another super antioxidant nutrient that's easily wiped out by smoking, traffic pollution and stress is vitamin C. Vital for fighting infection, for wound-healing and the formation of collagen (a protein essential for making ligaments, bones, teeth and the 'cement' that holds the skin together). Collagen degeneration can be linked to a lack of vitamin C; when the elasticity of collagen collapses, skin drags and sags. Vitamin C has hundreds of other biochemical tasks, too. It reduces the risk of arterial damage and cardiovascular disease, balances blood cholesterol, protects against stress, reduces allergic reactions and is needed for energy production. In fact, this most vital of vitamins is involved in around 300 different body processes. And even though there is no evidence that vitamin C can actually *cure* a cold, I know I'm not the only one who is convinced that taking extra C wards off infections *and* hastens healing.

Common signs of vitamin C deficiency:

Frequent colds/infections	Easy bruising
Bleeding gums	Cystitis
Constipation	Haemorrhoids (piles)
Broken capillaries	Cuts that won't heal
Clogged arteries	High cholesterol

Some doctors believe that it's a waste of time taking more vitamin C than the official Recommended Daily Amount (now called the RNI or Reference Nutrient Intake), because excesses will be wasted via the urine. But if you examine the research closely, the old argument about 'expensive urine' simply doesn't stand up.

Human beings are one of the few animal species no longer able to manufacture their own vitamin C; so we must get our supplies from what we eat. A number of leading experts now take the view that, although the recommended daily amount of 60 mg may prevent scurvy, it isn't nearly enough for optimum health. It seems that most people need levels far above the officially recommended amount before any vitamin C shows up in the urine. In addition, vitamin C protects the bowel, bladder and kidneys – so even that which does pass through is of benefit. And don't forget that any vitamin C that ends up in the urinary system has probably been working hard in other parts of the body before it gets there. Remember that vitamin C is water soluble and is not stored by the body, so needs to be replenished every day.

In the Know
You might have read or heard that vitamin C causes kidney stones. It's an old chestnut that keeps popping up, but has no scientific evidence to back it.

Need More C?
If you are a worrier, suffer from stress and anxiety, get lots of colds, are plagued with cystitis, work in a polluted atmosphere, smoke (or live, work or socialize regularly with other smokers), are surrounded by electrical and electronic equipment or travel regularly in heavy traffic, try supplementing your diet with 1 or 2 grams daily of vitamin C complex.

Look for labels on vitamin C Complex that say 'low acid' or 'buffered' ascorbates. Try Blackmores' Bio-C or Ester-C Plus from Solgar. They're usually gentler on the stomach. Brands that fizz in water or are pure ascorbic acid with no buffering may be too acidic and could upset a sensitive digestive system.

Don't rely on supplements alone. Make sure your diet contains lots of vitamin C-rich foods. Most fruits and vegetables contain some vitamin C, so aim for two or three pieces of fruit, a good helping of fresh vegetables and a salad every day.

Where to Find Vitamin C

Acerola cherries	Kiwi fruits
Apricots	Kohlrabi
Bell peppers	Kumquats
Blackcurrants	Lemons

Broccoli   Mustard and cress
Brussels sprouts   Papaya
Cabbage   Parsley
Cauliflower   Bell peppers
Grapefruit   Sweet potatoes
Green leafy vegetables   Tomatoes
Guava   Turnip tops
Jacket potatoes   Watercress
Kale

Flavonoids

Flavonoids are something to get very excited about because they are so important to skin health. They belong to a large group of water-soluble compounds which are found, along with vitamin C, in plant foods.

The strange-sounding *quercitin*, *rutin* and *hesperedin* which you see on some supplement labels, especially in vitamin C complex, are members of the flavonoid family. So, too, are the newer discoveries that provide the red, blue and purple pigments in bilberries, cranberries and grapes. Called *anthocyanadins* and *proanthocyanadins*, they have especially powerful antioxidant activity.

Signs that flavonoids might be lacking in your diet:

Broken veins   Easy bruising
Haemorrhoids (piles)   Varicose veins/ulcers
Unexplained nosebleeds   Bleeding gums/nosebleeds
Ulcers   Stomach acidity

Flavonoids have been found to be beneficial in the treatment of fluid retention, heavy menstrual bleeding, allergies, haemorrhage, diabetic retinopathy and high blood pressure. Some evidence suggests they may also be useful in treating fatigue and to protect against skin damage caused by UV rays. Their outstanding anti-inflammatory and antioxidant properties make them superlative skin nutrients in their own right, helping to maintain the integrity of blood vessels and capillaries, and reducing pain, bruising and bleeding. They protect against free radical attack, shield vitamin C from damage and enhance its favourable effects. Some kinds of flavonoids are able to adhere themselves to collagen fibres to offer additional defence and restore flexibility and resilience. Healthy collagen cannot be produced or repaired without it.

It's interesting to note that, half a century ago, flavonoids were produced and sold by leading pharmaceutical companies to treat haemorrhage and capillary fragility, but were withdrawn from sale because they were said to be ineffective. Research since that time has shown this decision to be exceedingly premature.

Where to Find Flavonoids

Apples	Cherries
Apricots	Cranberries
Beetroot	Grapes
Bell peppers	Green tea
Bilberries	Onions
Blackcurrants	Papaya
Broccoli	Red wine
Buckwheat	Pith and skin of citrus fruits
Cantaloupe melon	

! **In the Know**
The plant-based remedies silymarin (milk thistle), resveratrol (grape seed extract), ginkgo biloba and pycnogenol (pine bark extract) are all rich sources of flavonoids.

Vitamin D

It has long been known that vitamin D is an essential requirement for strong bones and teeth, but new research suggests that it may also play a part in improving bone density after the age at which bone growth is said to be completed: usually between the ages of 30 and 40. Vitamin D is found in foods such as oily fish and eggs and is also produced by the action of daylight on the skin – one of the reasons why it is so important to spend time out of doors even on overcast days. See page 110 for more on essential sun protection.

In one study, post-menopausal women who were given small amounts of additional vitamin D (equivalent to only one half-hour's sunlight exposure per day) showed a significant increase in bone strength. In another, winter-time bone loss was reduced and bone density improved in women who took vitamin D. In a third, increases in bone mineralization were demonstrated in subjects who took additional calcium in an easily assimilated form. Without vitamin D, calcium cannot be properly utilized within the body.

Like vitamin A, vitamin D can be toxic if you take too much. The small amounts included in good-quality multivitamin preparations are fine, but larger, separate supplements of vitamin D should only ever be used under a practitioner's supervision.

Where to Find Vitamin D

Cod liver oil	Salmon
Free-range eggs	Sardines
Mackerel	Tuna

and from sensible exposure to sunshine (see section on Sun Care page 105).

Vitamin E

Now scientifically proven in the prevention and treatment of heart disease and circulatory disorders, vitamin E is also *the* vitamin for reducing scarring following accident or surgery. It can even reduce the prominence of old scars if applied regularly, and has been used to help burn victims. Vitamin E is known to prolong cell life, improve skin quality, prevent blood-clotting and hasten wound-healing.

All kinds of skin conditions, from the very dry to the very oily, including eczema, acne, psoriasis, sunburn, scalds and stretch marks, can be helped by topical applications of vitamin E. I have found that the best way to apply vitamin E is to pierce a capsule with a sterilized needle and massage it gently and directly into the skin with clean fingers. Or add it to your moisturizer.

Extra vitamin E can be helpful where there is:

Dry skin	Scarring
Heart disease	High blood pressure
Hormonal imbalance	Easy bruising
Stress	Poor circulation

Vitamin E protects unsaturated fatty acids and other fat-soluble nutrients from attack by oxygen. When fats and oils are refined – or their chemical structure altered – vitamin E is destroyed, so if your diet is high in processed foods and hydrogenated spreads, you could benefit from taking additional vitamin E as a supplement. But avoid large doses, which are unnecessary and could be dangerous. A daily amount of 100 to 400 iu (as part of a multi-complex formula) will give good antioxidant protection.

Where to Find Vitamin E
In cold pressed oils, especially:

Cod liver oil   Soya bean
Extra virgin olive oil   Sunflower
Linseed oil   Rice Bran
Safflower

Also in:

Almonds   Free range eggs
Apples   Granola
Bananas   Onions
Broccoli   Potatoes
Brown rice   Salmon
Brussels sprouts   Seeds
Carrots   Spinach
Cashew nuts   Sprouted grains

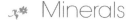 # Minerals

Calcium

Calcium has many roles in the body apart from being the major constituent in our teeth and bones. Without it, nerves would not function, skin and muscles would lack tone and strength, blood vessels would weaken and skin would not heal.

Calcium is also an important factor in the metabolism of essential fatty acids and – with vitamin C – in the manufacture of collagen, and it works closely with other nutrients to maintain healthy skin.

Calcium deficiency can lead to:

Bone pain	Depression
Slow healing and mending of fractures	Easily broken bones
	Panic attacks
Muscle spasms and twitching, particularly of the limbs	Insomnia

As with all minerals, absorption of calcium can be hampered by many factors:

☒ Too many saturated fats in the diet can form insoluble soaps with calcium in the body, so keep saturates to sensible limits.

☒ Rhubarb: apart from being uncomfortably acidic, it contains oxalates which bind to calcium and prevent its absorption.

☒ The phytates in unrefined grains do much the same thing, so steer clear of coarse wheat bran – the 'sawdust' sprinkled over breakfast cereals.

☒ Calcium doesn't like diets which contain too much phosphorus (found in red meat, carbonated drinks, junk food).

☒ Stomach acid is needed to dissolve calcium prior to absorption. If you experience persistent indigestion immediately after meals, you could be suffering from an under-acid stomach (hypochlorhydria), often mistaken for over-acidity.

☒ Excess use of aluminium-based antacids can prevent calcium absorption.

☒ Vitamin D (converted by the skin from daylight) is absolutely essential if calcium is to be properly utilized. Try to spend some time outdoors every day if possible.

☒ Diets high in animal protein cause calcium to be excreted in excess by the kidneys.

[X] Lactose intolerance – the inability to digest milk sugar – may prevent absorption of calcium from milk. But there are plenty of other calcium-rich foods to choose from (see below).

[X] Magnesium must be present for calcium to be properly assimilated, so it's important to include magnesium-containing nuts, wholegrains, fresh fruit and vegetables in the diet.

Milk is generally put forward as an A1 source of calcium. A terrifically nutritious food for calves, I have never believed that cow's milk is a natural food for humans. An infamous allergen, it is well known for causing indigestion, catarrh and a range of other symptoms, including skin eruptions in some sensitive individuals. However, milk can be useful as a topical cleanser and moisturizer.

You may enjoy drinking milk and suffer no side-effects. Small amounts in tea and coffee are less likely to present problems. However, if you're troubled by any of the above symptoms, you may find that it's better to avoid cow's milk and, instead, include lots of other foods rich in calcium.

Where to Find Calcium

Almonds	Pulses
Brazils	Root vegetables
Brown rice	Sea vegetables
Buttermilk	Sesame seeds
Canned salmon	Stock made with bones
Canned sardines	Sunflower seeds
Cheese	Tahini
Figs	Tofu
Green vegetables	Yoghurt
Oats	

An overload of calcium from individual supplements may do more harm than good if your diet is lacking in other balancing nutrients such as magnesium and vitamin D. This doesn't mean, however, that calcium is bad for us, far from it; simply that any nutrient swallowed in large amounts or as a separate supplement could be mishandled by the body and not work as it should.

> **In the Know**
> If you have a family history of osteoporosis or are worried about brittle bone disease, see your GP for a check-up and ask to be referred to a nutrition practitioner who can properly analyse your diet and your nutrient intake.

Chromium

It has been said that the total amount of chromium required by one human being for a whole lifetime would fill only an egg cup – and yet, because of intensive farming, crop spraying, food processing and high-sugar diets, this trace mineral is one of the most commonly deficient.

Essential for controlling blood glucose levels and for balancing blood fats and cholesterol, you could be short of chromium if you have:

Excessive thirst	Excessive sweating
Dizziness or poor concentration after more than three hours without eating	Need for frequent meals
Poor co-ordination	Waking hungry during the night
Night sweats	High blood fats and/or high cholesterol
Drowsiness during the day	Chronic fatigue or sudden unexplained exhaustion
Hypoglycaemia	Family history of diabetes

Where to Find Chromium

Asparagus	Plankton
Blackstrap molasses	Raw beetroot
Cheese	Seafood
Egg yolk	Spirulina
Lamb's liver	Wholegrains

By reducing the risk of hypoglycaemia and diabetes, good chromium levels also guard, indirectly, against nervous system damage such as diabetic neuropathy and may be helpful in reducing elevated blood fats (*triglycerides*) and high cholesterol.

Iron

Population studies carried out around the world would suggest that iron deficiency is extremely common. For example, an Australian dietary survey published in 1988 showed 45 per cent of women to be low in iron – and also in calcium, zinc, magnesium and vitamins A, C and B_6. A similar UK investigation of 800 people indicated that 60 per cent of women had iron intakes below the RDA. And things haven't changed much since then.

In food, iron exists in two different forms: organic *haem* iron is abundant in meat foods, from which it is generally well absorbed. Inorganic *non-haem* iron is the kind found in vegetables, fruits and nuts; it must be altered chemically by the body before it can be used, and cannot be absorbed without vitamin C. Mother Nature knows this, which is why iron and vitamin C are found together in so many fruits and vegetables. Malic acid, found in plums, apples and pumpkin, and the citric acid in citrus fruits, also enhance the absorption of this 'veggie' iron. Interestingly, iron deficiency appears to be rare in vegans and vegetarians, but widespread among the population as a whole.

Iron is an essential trace mineral needed to make haemoglobin – the red pigment in blood cells – and myoglobin, another iron-containing pigment which carries and stores oxygen in muscle tissue. Iron is also an important constituent in a number of enzymes, and is vital for healthy growth and mental development. If iron stores are low, the body will try to compensate by absorbing more from food, but when reserves fall too far the result is iron-deficiency anaemia.

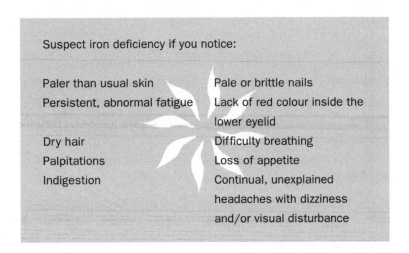

Suspect iron deficiency if you notice:

Paler than usual skin

Persistent, abnormal fatigue

Dry hair

Palpitations

Indigestion

Pale or brittle nails

Lack of red colour inside the lower eyelid

Difficulty breathing

Loss of appetite

Continual, unexplained headaches with dizziness and/or visual disturbance

Vitamin B$_{12}$ is essential for the absorption of iron and may be lacking if you are experiencing digestive discomfort, have a bright red tongue or suffer with nervous disorders, tingling in the fingers and toes or poor co-ordination. Iron absorption may also be inhibited where there is insufficient vitamin C, vitamin A, folic acid or copper or an excess of zinc. Problems of deficiency may be further aggravated by aspirin-based drugs, lack of stomach acid, too much cereal fibre in the diet or too many cups of tea or canned fizzy drinks.

Anyone concerned that they are anaemic or unable to consume enough iron should ask their doctor for a blood test before launching into self-prescribed iron tablets. Most types of iron supplement are notoriously poorly absorbed and well known for their gut-irritating and constipating talents – and overdosing on iron could be dangerous. If you have iron supplements in the house, keep them right away from youngsters. As little as 3 mg could kill a small child.

Where to Find Food Sources of Iron

Apples	Nuts
Bananas	Parsley
Beetroot	Pulses
Blackstrap molasses	Sardines
Broccoli	Seeds
Cabbage	Sweet potato
Celery	Tomatoes
Dried fruit	Turnip
Eggs	Watercress
Endive	Wholegrains
Lamb's liver	

Magnesium

Not only is magnesium a vital partner to calcium, it also assists the B vitamins and essential fatty acids, so is fundamental for healthy skin. It works to repair and maintain cells and tissues, balance hormones and support the nervous system.

If you are short of magnesium, you might notice symptoms such as:

Breathlessness	Constipation
Cramp	Depression or anxiety
Dizziness	Insomnia
Muscle spasm	Muscle weakness
Palpitations	Period problems
Poor co-ordination	Pre-menstrual syndrome
Restless limbs	Sweating
Twitchy muscles	Unexplained fatigue

! In the Know
Magnesium supplements have been found to be helpful in the treatment of Chronic Fatigue Syndrome and for reducing the risk of blood clots following surgery. Some experts are sure that magnesium could be even more important than calcium in the fight against brittle bone disease.

Where to Find Magnesium

Almonds	Haricot beans
Apples	Lemons
Bananas	Pasta
Brazils	Plankton
Brown rice	Pulses
Cashews	Seafoods
Dark green vegetables	Sesame seeds
Dried fruit, especially figs	Sprouted seeds
Grapefruit	Wholegrain flour
Green vegetables	

Many varieties of vegetables contain small but valuable amounts of this important skin mineral.

Selenium

A trace element, needed only in tiny quantities, selenium forms a vital part of the antioxidant enzyme glutathione peroxidase. The functions of selenium include the maintenance of healthy skin and hair, protection against free radical activity and pollution, as well as support for the immune system. Evidence shows that selenium is frequently deficient in patients with cancer, rheumatoid arthritis and heart disease; also that taking selenium supplements may help to reduce the risk of certain types of cancer. Selenium works synergistically with vitamins C and E, two other important antioxidant skin protectors; it also plays an important anti-inflammatory role in the body.

Selenium deficiency signs include:

Angina	Bleeding nails
Brittle, flaking nails	Dry, flaking skin
Hair, skin and nail problems	High blood pressure
Poor resistance to infection	Poor wound healing
Stiff and painful joints	

Where to Find Selenium

Fish and shellfish	**Milk**
Free-range eggs	**Wholegrains, especially brown rice**
Fruits and vegetables	

Unfortunately, soil deficiency of this mineral is common, which means that crops grown in poor soil are likewise low in selenium. Mounting evidence suggests that we all might benefit by taking a daily selenium supplement.

Zinc

The benefits which zinc bestows upon the skin should not be underestimated. Some experts believe zinc deficiency to be endemic – and my own experience with patients would certainly suggest that low zinc levels are extremely common, particularly where skin problems are concerned.

Without zinc, vitamin A cannot be properly utilized. Zinc is vital for growth and repair, for wound-healing, balancing insulin production and for helping other hormones.

Symptoms of zinc deficiency include:

Acne	Blood sugar disorders
Digestive problems	Excessively dry or excessively oily skin
Infertility	Loss of taste or smell
Persisting infections	Poor appetite
Poor hair quality	Slow wound-healing
White marks on the fingernails	

Where to Find Zinc

Cheese	Milk
Fish	Nuts
Free-range eggs	Plankton and other seaweeds
Grains	Pumpkin seeds
Kelp	Seafood
Meat	Vegetables

Even where the diet is well supplied, however, absorption can be poor because zinc competes with other minerals – such as calcium – for transport across the gut wall. Food additives can adversely affect the absorption of zinc, as can too much of the wrong kind of dietary fibre. For this reason it is probably wise to avoid wheat bran and wheat-based cereals, choosing wholegrain rye, rice, oats, buckwheat and millet instead.

In the Know
Research has proven that zinc gluconate lozenges, if sucked regularly at the first sign of cold symptoms, can reduce both the severity and the duration of the virus. Strangely, swallowing extra zinc supplements did not have the same effect.

Essential Fatty Acids

Remember we looked at these important nutrients when we were talking about fats and oils on page 25? Well, you'll also recall that EFAs have lots of vital functions and are especially important to skin health. They're needed for the structure of every cell membrane and play an important role in maintaining muscle tone, skin moisture and smoothness. EFAs also assist oxygen uptake and are an important component in energy production. And lack of them – wouldn't you just know it? – plays havoc with our hormones.

Essential fatty acids fall into two basic family groups, known as Omega 3 and Omega 6. They may sound similar but are needed for completely different tasks within the body. That's why it's so important to make sure that we eat foods regularly from both groups.

Omega 3 oils come from fatty fish such as mackerel, tuna, salmon and sardines – and they're found in linseeds and walnuts. You can also find Omega 3 in fish oil supplements (it's important to look for labels that tell you the EPA and DHA content – see below).

Omega 6 oils turn up in seeds, nuts, some vegetables and pulses, and in the cold-pressed oils that come from pumpkin and sunflower seeds, safflower, almonds, etc. Good quality supplements of evening primrose oil and borage oil provide Omega 6 in a specially converted form known as GLA (gamma linolenic acid).

EFAs get to be called essential because they can't be made inside the body and have to be provided, one way or another, by the diet.

But swallowing them isn't enough. Before the body can use them internally, enzymes are needed to alter the structure of essential fatty acids. Unfortunately, research suggests that quite a lot of people are unable to make this conversion and scientists suspect this may be just one of many reasons why deficiencies of these important nutrients appear to be on the increase. And that's where supplements could be of value, especially if they are used in conjunction with a healthy diet.

Supplementing with GLA and fish oils may help to overcome dietary deficiencies and give considerable relief to a range of diseases commonly associated with a lack of EFAs, including:

Eczema	Psoriasis
Mastalgia	Pre-menstrual syndrome
Heart and circulatory disorders	Viral infections
Post-viral fatigue	Multiple Sclerosis
Diabetes	

Hemp Seed Oil

If evening primrose was the oil of the 1980s and flax seed the nutritional news of the 1990s, then the miracle plant for the millennium could turn out to be hemp seed. Like linseed/flax, the oil from hemp seed is not only rich in GLA but provides an excellent ratio of Omega 6 to Omega 3 essential fatty acids, together with a worthwhile source of vitamin E, calcium, magnesium and potassium. Actual scientific research is still limited, but that hasn't stopped hemp seed oil being hailed as one of the best anti-cholesterols, widely recommended as healthy for the heart and the hormones. With an enviable anti-inflammatory, anti-allergic and anti-arthritic pedigree, its perfect fatty acid content makes it a super skin nutrient, feeding flexibility to cell membranes and boosting anti-viral, anti-fungal and anti-bacterial protection.

Tips

Hemp oil is often advertised with a long list of glowing adjectives. It isn't a miracle cure but may be a worthwhile dietary supplement, especially if you're suffering from unresolved dry – or oily – skin conditions, are distressed by eczema or psoriasis or have elevated cholesterol levels.

For best absorption, always take hemp seed oil with a meal. There is no need to take lots of different fatty acids supplements (i.e. fish oil, linseed/flax, GLA and hemp) all at the same time.

Hemp seed oil is available in capsule form from good health stores and from Viridian (see page 229 for stockist information).

Hemp seed oil comes with one major caution. There have been a few cases where hemp seed products in the diet, like poppy seeds on a bagel, have caused a false-positive result in a standard drug test. Although completely legal, non-toxic, non-addictive and without side-effects, hemp seed just happens to belong the Cannabis family. Study results concluded that 'commercially available cold-pressed hemp seed oil contains cannabinoids at levels capable of producing a positive workplace test for marijuana.' Recently, two court cases have overturned marijuana charges after weighing evidence that the defendants had consumed hemp oil. As its dietary use gains popularity, employers and officials need to be aware that this legal food product may make urine testing for cannabis unreliable, and that workplace testing procedures may need to change.

✳ Supplement Sense

If you decide to follow a course of supplements, here are a few tips:

✓ Don't supplement for the sake of it. If you are suffering from one of the conditions listed above or believe that essential fatty acids may help your particular health problem, I would very strongly recommend that you seek a consultation with a qualified practitioner who specializes in nutritional therapy and can properly assess your diet.

✓ Sort out your Omega families. If you're looking for Omega 3 fish oil supplements, check that they contain EPA and DHA. EPA stands for eicosapentaenoic acid; DHA for docosahexaenoic acid. You don't need to be bothered about these weird-sounding words, but if these particular letters aren't mentioned on the label, chances are the product you are looking at is not a particularly rich source of Omega 3 oils. If you eat oily fish twice a week, it may not be necessary to spend money on fish oil supplements as well.

✓ It's worth knowing that most cod liver oil supplements – although a rich source of vitamins A and D, and good for helping ease stiff joints and perhaps, reducing the risk of catching a cold – may be very low in the EPA and DHA content that's reputed to be helpful for such conditions as psoriasis.

✓ If you're looking for Omega 6, check labels for GLA (gamma linolenic acid). Find it in borage oil (also called starflower oil), blackcurrant seed oil, evening primrose oil and sometimes from herbal sources. The percentage of GLA per capsule is important, so again, if the label or product leaflet doesn't give that information, it may not contain sufficient GLA to help you.

✓ Top quality linseed (or flaxseed) oil contains appreciable amounts of both GLA and EPA, so it's a good one-stop compromise that is also suitable for vegetarians and vegans. However, beware of low-cost products which may not be pure or of the best quality.

✓ Buy the best that you can afford. (See my recommendations later in this section.) Cheaper supplements can seem like a good deal but may, in fact, be a false economy if they are poorly absorbed or too low a dose to make the difference.

✓ It's worth knowing that low doses for short periods of time probably may not have any significant effect; that's why it's important to take the recommended dose for at least three months before assessing any improvements.

✓ Keep supplements in a cool place, away from light. Linseed oil products should always be kept in the fridge.

✓ I would recommend Biocare, Pharma Nord and Solgar as some of the best for quality GLA and fish oil supplements. Linseed/flaxseed oil is available in capsule form from Biocare and from Viridian and in liquid form from Savant-Health (see Resources chapter).

> ! In the Know
> A capsule of evening primrose oil or GLA squeezed into a large dollop
> of unperfumed hand cream or body lotion makes a healing treatment
> for dry or chapped skin.

Probiotics

When looking at vital body nutrients, probiotics are an often-overlooked
factor. Yet they play an important role in maintaining the health of the
skin, have much-needed antioxidant capabilities and are a powerful force
in restoring the status quo after antibiotics. In some countries they are
prescribed routinely following antibiotics to help repopulate the gut.

These friendly flora of the digestive tract have many beneficial actions
in the healthy activity of the gut and are particularly important in the
maintenance of blooming skin. Apart from assisting in the process of
detoxification, their natural antibiotic activity helps to boost immunity,
inhibit the growth of undesirable bacteria and promote vitamin synthesis.

Repairing the Damage

One of the simplest and safest ways of restoring gut flora balance is to
reinstate the beneficial bacteria in the form of live yoghurt and probiotic
supplements. I cannot emphasize too strongly the importance of purchas-
ing only the best quality supplements. Check the label to make sure that
the capsules contain the right kinds of bacteria – *Lactobacillus acidophilus*
(which lives in the small intestine) and *Bifido bacterium* (which live in the
large bowel). Also, bear in mind that it can take several months to restore
the favourable habitat of the intestines (especially after long-term use of
antibiotics), so supplementation may need to be continued for several
months – accompanied, of course, by a varied and nourishing diet.

Live yoghurt alone is not always sufficient to repopulate the gut after
antibiotic ingestion. In addition, a number of yoghurts tested for their culture counts were not as 'alive-alive-o' as their packaging proclaimed.
While good quality bio-yoghurts are certainly beneficial (their lactic acid

content lowers the pH of the intestines and creates a more favourable environment for friendly bacteria to grow), not all the bacteria they contain are likely to survive the rigorous journey through the stomach.

Give them the best chance by buying yoghurts that are well before their 'use by' date (the older they get, the lower the culture count) and always store them carefully in the fridge. Avoid those that are flavoured and contain artificial additives.

To further encourage re-population of these beneficial bugs, probiotics in the form of supplements can be invaluable. Unfortunately, independent assays carried out around the world have shown that many of the probiotic products on the market simply do not contain the active friendly flora which the labels would suggest. It is therefore vital to choose only those which passed these tests with flying colours. My personal choice would be either Biocare's Replete or their Bio-Acidophilus capsules, or Blackmores' Acidophilus & Bifidus.

Are Dietary Supplements Important to Skin Health?

In an ideal, unpolluted world, obtaining all the goodness needed from diet alone might be a possibility. That is, of course, so long as that goodness is properly absorbed. Unfortunately, however, the perfect diet has become rather elusive. Adding a really good quality multivitamin/mineral, extra vitamin C and some essential fatty acids to your main meal of the day could make good health sense in our stressed and polluted world.

Nutritional supplements have an enviable safety record. Figures produced by the American Centers for Poison Control (they monitor drug safety data) estimate them to be 'at least 1,200 times safer than any drug' and, ultimately, following more research 'perhaps tens of thousands of times safer'.

Consider supplements if you suffer from:

Skin problems	Breaking nails
Excessively dry or oily hair	Heavy periods
High blood pressure	High cholesterol
Excessive stress, anxiety or panic attacks	Digestive and/or bowel problems
Persistent colds or other infections	

Or if you:

Smoke	Diet regularly
Drink huge amounts of tea, coffee or cola	Eat lots of sugary or fatty foods
Exist on take-aways or packets and tins	Travel frequently in heavy traffic
Work in a polluted atmosphere	Have been ill
Are waiting for an operation	Are just out of hospital
Are taking regular prescribed or over-the-counter medication, especially HRT, the contraceptive pill or regular doses of aluminium-based indigestion remedies	

And also if you are:

Vegetarian or vegan	Pregnant
Breast-feeding	

There remains an unfortunate tendency to besmirch and slander supplements, but a multitude of properly controlled scientific studies carried out around the world continue to show the power and protection that can be provided by natural food substances. Vitamins A, C and E, essential fatty acids, magnesium, calcium, chromium and selenium are just a few examples of nutrients which have been used in the treatment of a range of medical conditions from childhood measles, pre-menstrual syndrome and skin disorders to arthritis, heart disease and cancer, with some astonishing and exciting results.

My own experiences, both personally and with patients, have convinced me that supplements, if used sensibly, can be of enormous value in helping to prevent, treat and alleviate many different conditions and are of particular merit in overcoming skin disorders.

But the market is awash with thousands of different products; choosing the right supplements can be a minefield for the unwary. My supplement guidelines may help you to avoid the pitfalls:

* Don't be fooled by cheap products.
* If the label lacks detail, don't buy the product.
* The product should be free from gluten, yeast, colours, sugar, lactose, fillers, binders, corn, wheat, salt, preservatives, artificial flavours, milk and soy products (if it is, the label will tell you so); these are often added to save money, but can destroy the nutrients you want – and some are potential allergens.
* Check the 'sell by' or 'use by' date.
* Store in a cool, dark place.
* Replace the lid securely after each use.
* Take all supplements with meals, unless the label tells you specifically to take them on an empty stomach.
* Be sensible. Follow the pack instructions and never exceed the stated dose. More does not necessarily mean better!
* Don't be frightened by scaremongers who try to persuade you that taking supplements is dangerous or a waste of time. They haven't

read the latest research. Good quality products have an excellent safety record.

* The word 'supplement' means what it says. Vitamin and mineral capsules should not be viewed as meal replacements and are not substitutes for a nourishing and varied diet.

* There is no need to buy masses of different jars and bottles or lots of separate, isolated nutrients. A good basic supplement programme consists of:

> the best quality multivitamin/mineral complex you can afford; at least 1 (preferably 2) grams of vitamin C complex; GLA or evening primrose oil;

* fish oil or linseed oil capsules (if you are not eating oily fish, such as mackerel, trout, sardines and salmon, two or three times per week).

Probiotics are recommended where there has been exposure to antibiotics, in bowel and digestive disorders, poor immune function and where there are skin problems.

Very Important Note: If you are concerned about your health in any way, please consult your doctor without further delay. Supplements can be enormously helpful, but are not substitutes for qualified medical advice. If you are pregnant or are taking regular medication and would like to take supplements as well, it is advisable to let your doctor know.

Organics

The history of agrichemicals is littered with toxic substances that were considered safe and then consequently withdrawn when they were shown to be dangerous, long after doubts about their safety.

JOANNA BLYTHMAN, *THE FOOD WE EAT*

 ## Organic Advantages

Although I'm not suggesting that eating organically cures skin conditions, or that eating foods that are grown using agrichemicals cause any skin disease, my own *very* strong instinct would be always to take the organic option. Not only am I convinced that foods treated with chemical sprays definitely DO NOT suit *my* skin or my well-being in general, I've also seen some pretty amazing improvements in patients who swapped regular for organic foods. Such as ...

> ... the young mum who suffered severe skin rashes on her face and neck whenever she ate fruit. She tried washing the fruit, peeling it, reducing the quantity eaten, but always her skin flared up about three or four hours after eating apples or pears. When she opted for the organic alternative, her skin did not react. And ...

... how about the 35-year-old who suffered with huge red and inflamed boils all over his back when he ate battery-raised poultry and eggs, but was not affected when he ate organically raised products? Of course it's impossible to know which residues, if any, might have been the specific cause. Or ...

... the woman who suffered migraine every time she ate ordinary chocolate, but not when she ate organic chocolate. Also, I wonder if ...

... artificial additives may, in some circumstances, be the trigger for skin problems? I can recall a number of cases where skin rashes, blotches and itches cleared up when artificial colourings, preservatives and flavourings were avoided.

It could all be down to coincidence, of course. But until someone can convince me that organic foods are no better for me than the rest, then I'll 'go organic' whenever I can.

Skin health apart, there are a whole host of excellent reasons for going organic.

Seven Good Reasons for Eating Organic

1   **Higher Vitamin and Mineral Content**
    Organic food has been shown in many studies to contain more vitamins, nutrients and cancer-fighting antioxidants than non-organic food; in some cases, twice and three times the vitamin and mineral value of chemically raised 'equivalents'.

2   **Grown without the Use of Artificial Chemicals**
Organic systems aim to avoid the use of artificial chemicals, pesticides, herbicides, fungicides and fertilizers and to produce food without the routine use of antibiotics and growth-promoting drugs.

3   **Free from Genetic Modification**
Organic food is produced without GMOs, which are prohibited within the Soil Association Standards for organic food and farming.

4   **Healthier Animals**
Most people are aware that organic farming places great emphasis on animal welfare, allowing livestock access to fresh air and open spaces. But did you know that BSE, known as mad cow disease, has not been found in any herd under full organic management since the early 1980s?

5   **Healthier Farmers**
Organic farmers don't use organophosphates. Farmers who use organophosphates suffer from more psychiatric and nervous system disorders and loss of mental skills than those who are not exposed.

6   **Supports the Natural Eco-system**
Organic production is more sustainable and friendlier to the environment and wildlife. In fact, organically-managed farmland supports more wildlife (including birds) than chemically-managed land. Pesticide poisoning is known to be directly responsible for the deaths of thousands of birds each year.

7   **Organic Tastes Better!**
If none of this convinces you, why not go organic just because it tastes better? If you think this is an exaggeration, just do the carrot test. Take an organic and a non-organic carrot. Wash them both thoroughly before you eat one and then the other. Do you think they taste the same? I don't mean to influence you, but whenever I repeat this test, I never fail to notice a strange chemical 'aftertaste' in the non-organic carrot.

> **Buzzword**
> *Antioxidants* are those very important nutrients and enzymes which help to guard the cellular structure and reduce oxidation; in other words, wrinkling, ageing and general degeneration.

Crop Chemicals

Organophosphates

Organophosphates are neurotoxic chemicals, originally developed as nerve gases, which are today used as pesticides. They've been linked with a number of health concerns including osteoporosis, ME (Chronic Fatigue Syndrome) and other serious problems.

The researchers who discovered a connection between organophosphates and Chronic Fatigue Syndrome have also found that there is a long delay between the actual exposure to the pesticide and the onset of the illness. In other words, the date of diagnosis might be many years after the contact with the chemicals concerned.

Pesticides and Environment

Pesticides are chemical substances used to kill or control pests of the crawling and flying variety. They work by attacking the central nervous system of the creature concerned. Unfortunately, they can also destroy beneficial species, in turn devastating entire eco-systems. Pesticides are known to affect human health adversely, both through short-term occupational poisoning or chronic long-term illnesses such as Chronic Fatigue Syndrome.

Despite all the platitudes dished out by agrichemical company spokespersons, it can be difficult to agree with them that crop chemicals present no potentially serious hazard. In one toxological survey that looked at 426 commonly-used chemicals, 68 were found to be carcinogenic,

61 had the ability to mutate human genes, 35 were found to affect reproduction adversely and 93 caused skin irritations.

The quantity of synthetic pesticides dumped on the land each year is absolutely staggering. Just the annual US production exceeds 600,000 tons – and this figure doesn't include herbicides, fungicides, fertilizers and other crop chemicals. In the United Kingdom the estimated figure quoted is over 4.5 billion litres of pesticide annually.

And I think we should be really concerned by the news that biologists have linked a number of pesticides and hormone residues in the environment to feminization and infertility in male birds, alligators, fish and turtles. Studies show that even minuscule exposure to these chemicals, far less than is known to cause cancer, is sufficient to damage an animal's ability to reproduce successfully.

One of the maxims that justifies the organic choice for me is the one that says you can always rinse or remove a slug or a greenfly from your cabbage, but you can't wash out or 'pick off' systemic agrichemicals.

What Does Organic Really Mean?

There really is more to organic farming than just avoiding the use of chemical pesticides. The aim of organic growers is to achieve healthful and wholesome produce in the most environmentally-friendly way possible. They pay particular attention to the quality of the soil – the key to nutritious food – depending upon traditional methods of crop rotation which help to encourage fertility and natural weed and pest control.

Manufacturers, producers and processors of organic foods are required to maintain detailed records. This means that animal and vegetable produce is fully traceable from the farm or the production plant, through the point of sale, to the table. The word 'organic' is now legally defined and organic food production and processing strictly monitored. Organic standards are stringent and cover every aspect of registration and certification, production, permitted and non-permitted ingredients, processing, packaging and distribution. They are also concerned with environment and conservation. And organic farmers, food-processors and manufacturers are subject to both annual and random inspections.

How Do You Know It's Organic?

The easiest way to find out is to check the packaging for a symbol of certification. All organic food sold in shops has to be marked clearly with an appropriate certification label. The one with which we are probably most familiar is the Soil Association. Others include the Organic Food Federation, the Organic Farmers & Growers and the Biodynamic Agricultural Association, known as Demeter. The Government authority – the body that sets the basic standards and is in overall charge – is called the UK Register of Organic Food Standards or UKROFS.

Can't Afford Organic?

Many people dump the idea of buying organic because they see it costing extra. Yes, organic produce is often more expensive. One of the principal reasons is the crop rotation I mentioned earlier. Unlike chemically-dependent farmers, who often grow the same crop in the same ground year upon year, a good organic harvest relies on the ability to leave fields fallow ('rest' them and leave them empty of crops) for one or more years at a time, so that the soil has a chance to regenerate. Not having a field in use means that the farmer is not earning from it. Another reason is that, while chemically-dependent farming is geared to mass production and therefore lower costs, organic food tends to be produced by small companies and individual suppliers.

But, for the consumer, with a little careful planning food bills don't need to be higher. In our house, we keep nutrients up and cost down by eating less meat and by basing some meals each week on cheaper ingredients such as organic mixed pulses, basmati or brown rice, couscous, jacket potatoes and other fresh organic vegetables. When I checked in two major supermarkets, a vitamin-rich and additive-free fresh organic apple cost less than a packet of crisps, a bar of chocolate or a slice of sticky cake!

Organic foods are required to meet extremely high standards. The principles of organic farming are based on creating a healthy, living soil which in turn produces healthy plants and animals. In an interesting and revealing study reported in 2001, public health experts who tested 3,200 organic vegetables found no evidence of four key microbes, *listeria, salmonella, campylobacter* and *E.coli* 0157, that might cause disease in humans. All the vegetables, which included lettuces, spring onions and carrots, were grown close to or in contact with the soil and sold for consumption without any further cooking.

By going organic you will be better nourished and may even save on bills as your shopping trolley loses those heavily processed and packaged non-organic items. Your skin will definitely thank you for the shift towards a simpler, purer diet.

Where to Buy Organic Food

Organic food is available through a wide range of outlets, including health stores and supermarkets. Direct-marketing schemes include farm shops, farm-gate and box schemes and farmers' markets.

Box Schemes
These have taken off in a spectacular fashion in the last few years. There are a number of different models, but all are based around the central principle of delivering a box of fresh, seasonal organic food, either directly to your door or to a central drop-off point.

Farm Shops, Farm-gate Sales and Farmers' Markets
For those within easy reach, all these offer the opportunity to buy fresh organic food directly from the producer. Some farm shops will buy in produce to supplement what they grow themselves. Again, many farm shops will keep regular customers in touch through newsletters and open days,

to help build up a loyal following. Farmers' markets – also on the increase – sell locally-produced goods and are an excellent source of affordable organic produce.

Supermarkets and Independent Retailers

All the large supermarket chains are now developing their organic food ranges. In addition there are an increasing number of independent retailers specializing in organic products, not only fresh food but also a wide range of dairy products, bakery goods and other processed foods and drinks.

As a result of the groundswell against genetically-modified foods, most supermarkets now stock a wider than ever range of affordable organic produce. However, if you think your food supplier is not stocking what you need, don't be afraid to ask. Store managers and owners will nearly always do whatever they can to stock new lines and that applies to organics too.

Independent Health Food Stores

Most independent health food retailers include an excellent range of organic and additive-free produce on their shelves.

The Organic Directory

If you're not sure where to find organic produce, invest in a copy of *The Organic Directory*, available from the Soil Association in book form at £7.95 plus postage, or find the same information for free on their website. It includes a comprehensive listing of organic suppliers, including box schemes and home delivery services, as well as providing information on organic B & Bs and restaurants.

Useful Organic Reading

Something else that 'did it for me' was reading *The Killing of the Countryside* by Graham Harvey (published by Jonathan Cape). This is a brilliantly researched account of how chemical warfare and other damage wrought to the countryside by modern farming practices is destroying the natural balance of nature. I recommend this book to everyone and I definitely recommend it to you. Another eye-opening book, *The Food We Eat* by Joanna Blythman (Michael Joseph), has an excellent section on chemically-dependent farming and organic alternatives and how to avoid pesticide residues. Highly recommended.

If you're looking for a really great organic cookbook, take a look at the *Organic Café Cookbook* by Carol Charlton. Beautifully illustrated, deliciously simple, scrumptious recipes.

And can I just say a final word on eating organically?

I think it's worth remembering that
what we do to our bodies,
we are bound to do to our skin.

I'd like to express my grateful thanks to the Soil Association for the information and reference material they have provided for this chapter.

part 2
··············

Detox

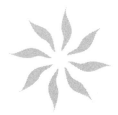

chapter 4

Good Digestion

I am convinced digestion is the great secret of life.

SYDNEY SMITH (1771–1845),

ENGLISH CLERGYMAN, ESSAYIST AND RENOWNED WIT

There seems little point in making any effort to improve the quality of food in our diet if no effort is made to improve the quality of digestion and absorption. Otherwise, nutrients are likely to be wasted. Healthy skin depends upon a constant supply of top-class nutrients – so making sure that those vitamins and minerals get to where they are needed is crucially important for skin health.

The following recommendations are all intended to help improve your intake of nutrients and the way your body digests and absorbs the food you eat. Don't be daunted by this list. No one is suggesting that you intro-duce everything all at once. Just take it easy, work through it, and try to make one or two changes each week or each month.

❋ Make time to eat regular meals, sit down to them and don't leave the table immediately to clear or wash the dishes; rest a while after eating. Never eat 'on the hoof'.

❋ Digestion begins in the mouth – that's what your teeth and saliva are for. The more chewing you do, the less churning further down the tubes and the more efficient the digestion. It sounds like common sense, but how many people do you know who *don't* bolt their food?

❋ Don't talk with your mouth full. This may seem a cheeky remark, but it is sensible. If you talk while you are chewing, you don't chew efficiently – *and* you swallow a lot of air which then rumbles around in the nether regions, interfering with proper digestion!

❋ Don't drink large amounts of fluid with meals. Small amounts – say a glass or a cupful – is fine.

❋ Drink plenty of water (preferably filtered) between meals, and carry water with you if you are travelling. Small bottles of water fit neatly into a bag, bottle-holder or car door pocket.

❋ Cut down on tea, coffee and other caffeine-rich drinks such as cola and hot chocolate. Instead, experiment until you find a herbal or fruit tea, grain-based coffee substitute or fresh fruit or vegetable juice you really like.

❋ Don't go for long periods of time without eating. If you know you are likely to miss a meal and will be hungry, take a snack with you and find a quiet spot to settle down and enjoy it without being rushed.

❋ Keep all fruits and fruit juices away from other foods. Enjoy them as in-between meal snacks and drinks, or as starters, but not with a meal – and certainly NEVER *after* a meal as a dessert.

❋ When eating out go for simple dishes and pass on the rich sauces or complicated menus.

❋ At home, don't deep-fry anything. Grill, bake, steam or stir-fry.

❋ Eat when you are hungry. Don't be forced into food just because the clock tells you it's time to eat.

❋ Always have breakfast, even if you can only manage a piece of fresh fruit and a glass of water. Remember that toast and coffee are both very acid-forming foods which can irritate the digestion, especially if you're rushed and stressed.

❋ Avoid reheats, except in emergencies. Reheating not only impairs flavour but also disturbs digestion and destroys nutrients. Stored cooked food, even when kept cool, can breed bacteria. If reheating is unavoidable, make sure that the meal is hot right through before serving and never reheat anything more than once.

❋ Introduce a small raw salad or selection of crudités 10 to 15 minutes before a cooked meal. The natural enzymes in the raw food not only help to enhance the digestion of the cooked meal which follows, but can also reduce the risk of overeating.

❋ If you are stressed, anxious or overtired but still need to eat, go for something light such as a salad or nourishing soup, rather than a heavy meal.

❋ Wash all fruits and vegetables thoroughly before use and avoid eating fruit skins unless you are sure that they are organically grown.

❋ Don't eat foods that are very hot or very cold. Remember that the stomach evolved long before cookers and refrigerators.

❋ Do what you can to cut right back on packaged, tinned, convenience and take-away foods which contain excessive amounts of refined flour, refined sugar, salt or spices (e.g. curries, chilli, etc.).

❋ Keep bread and wheat-based cereals to a minimum. Avoid white bread completely.

❋ Watch out for aluminium in the diet – it can disturb digestion. You'll find it in some kettles, cooking pots and utensils, toothpastes, dried milks, dried soups, coffee creamers, processed cheeses, cartoned juices, cigarette filters, table salt and a wide variety of prescribed medicines, particularly antacid indigestion remedies. Excesses of aluminium can disturb the balance of nutritional minerals in the body such as calcium and magnesium – both essential for healthy skin.

❋ Set realistic goals for yourself. Don't pursue a particular diet which you hate and which makes you miserable just because you have been told it is good for you.

❋ Include plenty of variety in your daily diet; be moderate and avoid excesses and extremes.

❋ Choose food that is as close to its fresh, natural state as possible.

❋ Adopt the easy-to-follow principles set out in my books *The Food Combining Diet* or *The Complete Book of Food Combining*, which involve:

   ❋ not mixing starch foods or sugars with proteins at the same meal

   ❋ keeping fruit away from proteins and starches.

After a few weeks of following this wonderful way of eating, any digestive discomfort should be a thing of the past and absorption and nutrient transport will improve – all vital for helping to improve the health of your skin.

5

Detox

There is no life without water ... Water is part and parcel of living machinery.

ALBERT VON NAGYRAPOLT SZENT-GYORGI,
POLISH SCIENTIST AND THE MAN WHO ISOLATED VITAMIN C IN 1922

Spring-cleaning Your Skin, from the Inside ...

If you've always steered clear of the word 'detox' because you thought it had to do with time-consuming diets or a restricted food intake and a generally pleasure-free existence, then think again. Detox is really all about cleaning up your diet, giving your digestion a break and giving your body the chance to shed some unwanted wastes. Done regularly, it not only cleanses the body but also sharpens the mind – and works wonders for the skin.

Fed up with excessive oiliness or dry flakiness? Puzzled by pimples, blotches and spots or that almost indefinable and yet obvious roughness or greyish pallor? All these can be signs of a skin under strain.

Toxicity can be a major handicap to improving skin quality – but short bouts of rest and relaxation, coupled with invigorating, cleansing skin foods and purifying fluids, can scrub your toxic tissues back to life and give your system a completely fresh start.

Detox can't cure pollution, of course. Dirt and grime don't disappear forever from your home just because you wash the kitchen floor or clean the windows. But in the same way that regular domestic cleaning reduces build-up, so regular detoxification helps the body's major routes of elimination – the lungs, the lymphatic system, the kidneys, liver, large intestine and, of course, the skin – to work more efficiently.

If you're interested in shedding a few pounds, detox can also kick stubborn weight problems into touch.

Poisons All Around Us

The human body accumulates poisons from lots of different sources, including:

- prescribed and 'social' drugs
- cigarette smoke
- alcohol
- industrial pollution
- vapours from household cleaning products
- poor quality diet
- food additives
- pesticides
- herbicides
- fungicides
- vehicle exhausts
- internal metabolic wastes.

Quite a list, isn't it? The system appears to cope, but is still likely to be stretched to the limits, especially when other stressors are added – for example anxiety, tension, worry, exhaustion, overwork, missed meals and so on.

When the body is on overload, we may put the red warning signals down to nothing more than 'feeling under par', little realizing that it could take just one more straw to break the camel's back!

Looking After Your Liver

The liver works particularly hard for us, but we treat it with very little respect. A massive filter with over 50 miles of tiny tubing, it screens heavy metals such as aluminium, lead, mercury and cadmium and is responsible for keeping the bloodstream free of potential poisons. Did you know that it filters, cleans and recycles 1 litre (2 pints) of blood every single minute of your life, sifting out and deactivating all kinds of metabolic wastes left-over from natural body functions as well as residues from things that we swallow or breathe in?

The only difference between someone who appears to 'get away with it' and another who shows symptoms of toxicity is whether or not the system can cope with the toxic loading without being damaged and still retain sufficient capacity to do other jobs. Don't forget that, in addition to all that cleaning up, your poor old liver has also to help control blood glucose, to regulate protein levels, to assimilate fats and control hormonal activity. And when symptoms do begin to develop, they may not necessarily show up in any orthodox medical test.

When we reach toxic overload, our skin, hair and nails are likely to be the first areas to register sapped energy and struggling life-force. The skin takes a lot of the strain as it tries to make up for the various inefficiencies of the other overworked organs. Chronic fatigue becomes more than a wearying nuisance and recurring infections and other illnesses grow more frequent.

Loving Your Lymph

Another area of the body that benefits hugely from a regular detox is the garbage collector known as the lymphatic system. An elaborate network of tiny tubes, not unlike blood capillaries, collects excess fluid, cellular debris and other unwanted material from the tissues, ready for discharge into the bloodstream.

And the lymph system isn't just about wastes. It is also an important route for transporting nutrients around the body.

If you suffer with swollen ankles, cellulite, breast tenderness, puffiness or dark circles around the eyes, persistent lethargy or seem to be plagued with a permanent cold or other infections, then your lymph system might be trying to tell you something.

Resting Your Digestion

Spring-cleaning the inside also means giving your intestines a bit of a holiday. Because most bodies are bombarded by constant supplies of food – often processed, refined and full of fats, sugars, salt, spices and stimulants – the digestive system is on permanent overtime. Giving it a rest allows every organ, gland, tissue and cell the chance to relax, unwind, cleanse and recharge.

It also makes sense to look after your digestion even when you are *not* detoxing. Find out how by checking out the section on the importance of good digestion on page 79.

Lifting Away the Lethargy!

Choose a couple of days when you are going to be at home. Weekdays or weekends, it doesn't matter. Just make sure that it's a time when you can be sure of some peace and quiet and are not under pressure from other people. When you find out how much you enjoy your detox days, I hope you will be able to make them a regular part of your routine; how about once a month? Just make it your quiet time. If you really feel that you can't manage a two-day break right now, at least try to complete Day One, and then repeat that day again in a couple of weeks' time.

Before you begin, read right through the following section so that you can make a shopping list of items you'll need.

This is a favourite detox diet that I hope you enjoy using:

First Things First
- ✓ Rest and relax as much as you can.
- ✓ Take a walk in the fresh air on both days, but don't play any sports, do workouts or undertake any other kind of strenuous exercise. Definitely don't walk or run near fume-laden traffic!
- ✓ Practise the deep breathing exercises detailed on page 184.
- ✓ For these two days, avoid all meat, poultry, fish, soya beans, cheese, alcohol, coffee, tea, sugar, bread, cereals, meals or snacks out of packets, carry-outs and take-aways. Instead, stick to fresh vegetables, juices and fruit.
- ✓ Ignore set meal-times during the detox. If you're hungry, eat some fresh or dried fruit, seeds, sheep's or goat's yoghurt, home-made soup or juice.
- ✓ Keep your fluid intake high. Drink plenty of freshly filtered water and vegetable juices throughout the day, to get those toxins moving and encourage a sluggish bowel back to life.
- ✓ Don't follow the cleansing routine for more than two or three days at a time or more than once in every two weeks.
- ✓ Look out those magazines, videos or that book you've been meaning to read for ages. Now's your chance to enjoy them.

Good Signs
If you've never followed any detox plan before this, don't be surprised if you notice mild symptoms such as a headache, slight nausea, a heavily coated tongue, catarrh or strong-smelling urine. You might find that you empty your bowels more frequently. Some people say that they experience bad breath, body odour, yawning and fatigue. All these are signs that the cleansing process is working. Try not to take painkillers or antacids to remove the symptoms of headache or indigestion, as drugs put further strain on the liver, encouraging toxins to go back into the tissues and thereby reversing the beneficial elimination process. As you detox more regularly, these signs should diminish.

> **In the Know**
> If your doctor or hospital has prescribed a special diet for you, if you have diabetes, are pregnant or on permanent medication for any condition or if you suffer from an eating disorder such as bulimia or anorexia nervosa, check with your GP before following this programme.

Day 1

ON WAKING
Practise one of the deep breathing exercises set out on page 184. Done regularly these exercises help to strengthen the lungs, improve the exchange of carbon dioxide and oxygen and enhance the transport of nutrients around the body.

ON RISING
Begin every day with a glass of boiled, cooled water livened up with a squeeze of fresh lemon juice. This is a wonderful skin cleanser and tonic. If you have a sweet tooth and find this mix too sharp, then add half a teaspoon of Manuka honey. Alternatively, enjoy a large cup of herbal tea with lemon juice or a glass of filtered water. Or if you have a juicing machine, blend your own favourite combination of fresh fruits.

BREAKFAST
Choose any fresh fruit and eat as much as you like. Mixed fruit salads are a great breakfast meal and surprisingly filling. How about a kiwi fruit, an apple and a nectarine? Or a ripe pear with a generous bunch of grapes? Or treat yourself to a whole mango or papaya? Anything goes – but please make sure you eat enough. One piece of fruit won't keep you going for long.

FRUITS TO CHOOSE
Apples, apricots (include soaked Hunza apricots, but avoid dried apricots if they are glazed or preserved), bananas, cherries, blackberries, blueberries, dates, figs, grapefruit, grapes, kiwi fruit, mango, nectarine, peaches, pears, pineapple, raspberries.

MID-MORNING BREAK

A cup of herbal tea, glass of fresh juice (not packaged orange juice) or water, a handful of mixed sunflower or pumpkin seeds and three or four dried figs. Dried figs are a wonderful source of dietary fibre and a terrific sweet treat. Just remove the tiny tough stalk and chew the fruit.

LUNCH/EVENING MEAL

Make either a large bowl of salad, a super stir-fry, vegetable compôte or a hearty home-made vegetable soup. Choose as many ingredients as you like from the boxes below.

For the soup, simply wash and chop vegetables into even-sized chunks, cover with filtered water, cook until tender and either mash or blend to a chunky or smooth liquid.

For the salad, chop, slice or grate your ingredients. Toss in a dressing of extra virgin olive and lemon juice, or leave plain.

For the stir-fry, heat the olive oil in a wok or pan. Fry crushed garlic and ginger for one minute. Add carrots, celery, broccoli florets, sliced bell peppers, spring onions, mangetout and courgettes. Cook for a further 3 to 4 minutes. Then add sprouts, sunflower and pumpkin seeds, and spinach leaves. Turn a few times to mix the ingredients. Serve immediately.

For the vegetable compôte, prepare your chosen vegetables into evenly-sized pieces or slices. Place all the ingredients into a steamer (or use a pan with a tight-fitting lid so that you add the minimum amount of water) and cook until just tender. Serve on its own with a little butter or a dressing made from extra virgin olive oil, cider vinegar and a twist of black pepper.

FOR A DELICIOUS STIR-FRY, CHOOSE FROM	FOR THE VEGETABLE COMPÔTE, CHOOSE FROM
Finely sliced celery	Broccoli florets (and stalks if they are young and tender)
Grated carrot	Brussels sprouts
Broccoli florets broken into small pieces	Carrot
Finely sliced bell peppers	Cauliflower florets (as for broccoli)
Finely sliced spring onions	Celery
Sliced green beans	Cabbage
Grated courgette	Courgette
Any sprouted beans or seeds	Leek
Half a teaspoon of grated root ginger	Onion
A handful of baby spinach leaves	Any kind of green beans
FOR VERSATILE VEGETABLE SOUPS, CHOOSE FROM	**FOR SCRUMPTIOUS SALADS, CHOOSE FROM**
Bell peppers	Avocado pear
Broccoli	Bean sprouts
Carrot	Raw grated beetroot
Cauliflower	Celery hearts
Cauliflower greens	Chicory leaves
Celery	Cucumber (skinned)
Leeks	Dark leaf lettuce
Onions	Red or white cabbage – finely sliced

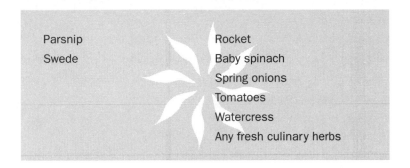

Parsnip
Swede

Rocket
Baby spinach
Spring onions
Tomatoes
Watercress
Any fresh culinary herbs

ALTERNATIVE SALADS

※ Grated raw beetroot and carrot with chopped onion, parsley and extra virgin olive oil and cider vinegar dressing

※ Grated carrot and apple with chopped celery and almonds

※ Fenugreek seeds with grated raw garlic, watercress, any grated cabbage, chopped cucumber and pine nuts, dressed with extra virgin olive oil and fresh lemon juice

※ Avocado slices with pumpkin seeds

※ Sliced apple with dried figs and hazelnuts

※ Skinned, sliced tomatoes with chopped basil, parsley and safflower oil

※ Broccoli or cauliflower florets dressed with hazelnut oil, cider vinegar and grated Brazils

Reminder
Buy organic produce whenever possible and remember to wash all produce thoroughly before use.

MID-AFTERNOON BREAK
A glass of juice or water and 2 teaspoonsful of organic linseeds. Just put one teaspoon of seeds at a time in your mouth and then several mouthfuls of fluid. The seeds will simply slide down your throat.

> **In the Know**
> Organic linseeds are available from good health stores. They're an excellent source of both soluble and insoluble fibre. They're one of the best remedies for constipation, but also said to be soothing and balancing for diarrhoea and irritable bowel.

AN HOUR BEFORE BED
Small carton of fresh plain full fat yoghurt (sheep's or goat's milk), followed by a cup of chamomile tea and honey.

Day 2
For breakfast, lunch and all snacks today, use liquids only, choosing from a variety of vegetable and fruit juices (preferably prepared at home from fresh produce) – drink any quantity you like. For your evening meal today, include a portion of brown rice with salad or steamed or stir-fried vegetables.

> **Buzzword**
> *Fasting*. A fast means eating no solid foods and surviving on water only for a period of days or weeks. It is not the same thing as a simple detox diet. Unless you are very experienced and know exactly what you are doing, fasting should only be carried out if supervised by a qualified practitioner.

Feeling Jaded? Try Juicing

Juicing has been around for many years and is synonymous with good health and longevity. Daily juicing was the mainstay of famous American naturopaths and physicians such as Benedict Lust and Dr Norman Walker, the latter a recognized authority on nutrition who lived for many hale and hearty years past his century. Some bookshops still carry copies of his classic paperback, *Fresh Vegetable and Fruit Juices* – well worth sleuthing for. And for sheer colour and exuberance, you could do no better than invest in a copy of *Super Juice* by Michael Van Straten. It's packed with the most delicious recipes.

Freshly prepared juices are a real health bonus. Made at home from delicious fruits and vegetables and using a simple juicing machine, they are also great energy-boosters and likely to be far more valuable nutritionally than those in bottles or cartons. The regular addition of raw juices to the diet will strengthen body function, providing the body with vital elements for repairing, renewing and revitalizing, encouraging the elimination of wastes and improving skin quality. They also have an amazing effect on a sluggish or irritable bowel and can (literally!) get you going in the morning.

Juices make nourishing sustainers for detox days and can provide essential nourishment during illness when solid foods may not be suitable or acceptable. And use them any time for super snacks or aperitifs.

All you need to try home-prepared juices for yourself is a juicing machine (available from most good electrical and hardware stores) and lots of fresh fruits and vegetables. Go for fresh fruit juice as a morning wake-up drink or pre-lunch appetizer and a vegetable juice medley prior to the evening meal. For best absorption, take them on an empty stomach – not with the meal. Soon you'll become really inventive with your recipes, producing colourful and flavourful combinations.

Just wash and peel the fruits and vegetables (no need to peel grapes!), push the pieces into the machine and let the equipment do the rest. In a couple of minutes you'll have a glass of wonderfully energizing fluid packed with vitamins, minerals and natural enzymes.

Go tropical and try fresh pineapple with mango, kiwi and papaya, apple and pear or nectarine with grape. Make a particularly cleansing and tasty aperitif with apple, celery, carrot, grape and beetroot (raw, not cooked).

Wonderful Water – The Skin Essential

French surgeon Dr Alexis Carrel was postulating the importance of water as a health-giver in the early 1900s and was awarded the Nobel Prize for

Medicine in 1912. 'The cell is immortal,' he said. 'It is merely the fluid in which it floats which degenerates. Renew this fluid at proper intervals, give the cells what they require for nutrition and, as far as we know, the . pulsation of life may go on for ever.'

Water is an essential part of your detox programme, but is also important at all other times, too. It's vital for skin health and beneficial for all skin types. A mere 2 per cent reduction of extra-cellular water can decrease energy levels by as much as one-fifth and can impair every single aspect of our bodily functions. Too little fluid can cause poor elimination of wastes, aggravate constipation and lead to urinary tract infections, particularly cystitis.

On other pages of this book I've looked at significance and value of the right kinds of fats, oils and fatty acids in achieving and maintaining glowing, healthy skin – but without sufficient water the body is unable to metabolize these important nutrients.

At birth the human body is made up of 90 per cent water, but on reaching adulthood this level drops to around 60 per cent. As we age the body 'tightens', cells begin to suffocate and die in their own waste products, metabolic 'trash' is not eliminated and the lymph system becomes overloaded. Water is needed to dilute the dross and debris so that they can be eliminated from the body. It plays a part in renewing cellular fluids, washing away the garbage and encouraging cell renewal, thereby reducing the effects of wrinkling and ageing.

Unless you are lucky enough to live in an area that has exceptional drinking water quality (and by that I mean that it doesn't smell like a swimming pool when you run the bath), filtered water is probably a good option. A quality filter unit should take out heavy metals such as lead, aluminium and cadmium plus chlorine and nitrates without disturbing the important nutritional minerals such as calcium. Write to manufacturers and seek out independent test results before you buy. Don't rely on the salesman's hype!

Water from a good-quality filter is also much cheaper than bottled water. Use it for cooking and filling the kettle too. Bottled water makes a good standby, especially if you are away from home, but choose those that are labelled 'low sodium'; many brands are high in salt, which can disturb potassium balance in the body as well as being drying to the skin.

In addition to any juice, coffee, tea or other beverages, try to drink a litre of water (approximately 2 pints) each day. This isn't difficult if you have a glass of water 10 to 15 minutes before each meal and keep another glass nearby to sip during the day. At work, give the vending machine a miss and drink water instead. Excessive amounts of coffee and tea overtax the liver and kidneys and rob the body of nutritional minerals, but unless your skin problem is very severe or food tests show them to be a factor, it shouldn't be necessary to give up tea and coffee altogether. Quality tea and coffee is often lower in caffeine than the cheaper varieties. Small amounts – say 1 to 3 cups daily – can be beneficial. If you are trying to cut down on caffeine, experiment with herbal teas, grain-based coffee substitutes, dandelion coffee, juices, clear soups or savoury herbal drinks.

... And from the Outside!

Bath twice a day to be really clean, once a day to be passably clean, once a week to avoid being a public menace.

ANTHONY BURGESS (1917–99), *INSIDE MR ENDERBY* (1963)

Cleansing

Cleaning the outside skin isn't just down to cleansing lotions or soap and water. You owe yourself more than that. Real cleansing means preventing those pores from choking to death, sloughing off dead cells, eliminating impurities and allowing your skin to 'breathe' and renew itself more efficiently. Don't forget that the skin – along with the bowel, bladder, kidneys, lungs and lymph system – is an important 'organ of elimination', and that when one area is sluggish the others will try to share the load. By making sure that the skin is functioning properly, other parts of the body will begin to work more efficiently, too.

Skin Airing

An 'old-fashioned' method of exposing the skin to fresh air is quoted almost lyrically by the famous 1930s fitness expert Mrs Mary M Bagot Stack in her book *Building The Body Beautiful – The Bagot Stack Stretch and Swing System* – now a collector's item. 'First thing, then,' she tells us, 'every morning, spring out of bed before you have time to hesitate or start that long line of thought which leads nowhere; throw open the windows. At first wear a bathing-dress and five jumpers if you feel the cold. But as your circulation improves each day, wear less and less, until finally your last bit of discarded silk or muslin can go across the window for the sake of the neighbours, but not around you!' Mrs Bagot Stack's suggestions of more than half a century ago may seem amusing and quaint, but were followed by millions of dedicated ladies at the time. Long before its association with the world-famous tenor, Luciano Pavarotti, gatherings of 10,000 or more would attend regular rallies in London's Hyde Park – all in the appropriate workout gear of the day – to follow Mary's exercise and breathing directions.

If the Bagot Stack experience is anything to go by, allowing unclothed skin to 'air' and practising your deep breathing exercises, especially near an open window, really will help to kick-start a sleepy body in the morning. It takes courage to begin with, but the long-term benefits are really worthwhile, especially if you are likely to be spending the rest of the day indoors!

Bathing

The word which usually springs to mind when we talk about the need for bathing or showering is 'cleanliness'. But a little extra time spent in the bath or shower than our usual daily dash can bring with it enormous health benefits and improvements to skin quality.

In the early 1900s, keeping clean was not so simple. Public bathing was more commonplace than it is now, each public bath (in London, at least) serving around 2,000 people! Few houses had indoor plumbing and, where a bathroom was boasted, it was usually of the cold comfort variety. But most modern dwellings have bathrooms luxurious enough to make relaxation a pleasure. So if you are an 'in-and-outer', slow down. Your health and your skin could benefit.

Skin Brushing

Brushing the hair is normal enough but, if you have never heard of it before, brushing the skin can seem a strange suggestion – until you realize what good sense it makes.

The health of the skin is determined to a great degree by its ability to repair and replace itself. If dead cells are not removed, pores can become clogged and congested. Where elimination is sluggish, new cells cannot work their way to the surface or may not be manufactured in the first place – and so damaged skin cannot heal. While skin cells are shed constantly (90 per cent of all household dust is said to be discarded human skin particles!), skin brushing stimulates the process into more efficient action. Circulation is improved, impurities are released and skin is healthier and softer.

The best and most effective skin brushes are made from natural materials and are usually used dry, before bathing. However, some ultra-sensitive skins may be more suited to wet brushing or to a loofah or bath mitt.

Here's how to do it:

Focus your movements towards the heart. Work your way from the soles of your feet, up your legs (remembering to brush the back of them as well as the front), over your thighs, buttocks, hips and torso, then up your arms towards your shoulders. Avoid the face but include the back of your neck. However, don't strain to reach the inaccessible parts of your back. And be gentle!

Other Effective Exfoliators

If brushing is difficult for you or for some reason not possible, stroke the skin firmly with an old and rough flannel face cloth, dry or wet. Damp cosmetic sponges (use a clean one each time) are good for the face and can be used with cleansers, scrubs and moisturizers. Or choose a body-scrub cream or lotion which you can massage into wet skin and rinse off in the bath or shower. A further option is to use a handful of oatmeal mixed to a paste with a teaspoon of jojoba oil and two drops of essential oil of juniper. Massaged into the skin before bathing or showering, this combination helps to detoxify, cleanse and moisturize the skin all in one go.

For very hard skin – on the heels or elbows, for example – rub with a handful of dry sea salt before bathing. Then, after drying the skin, apply this remedy: mix 2 drops each of lemon grass and lavender essential oils with 5 ml of almond oil. Massage the mixture well into the feet and elbows (the hands and nails are included automatically!).

If your skin is so sensitive that it reacts to even the word 'hypoallergenic', try a scrub of organic oatmeal followed by an oil blend of 5 ml of jojoba with 2 drops of chamomile and 2 drops of juniper essential oil.

How Often Should I Skin Brush?

After you have been skin brushing for a few weeks you will recognize automatically when it needs to be done. Since the gentle friction of brushing, loofahing and scrubbing actually cleanses the skin, I would recommend it every two to three days if you are showering or bathing every day. Brush every day if you shower or bathe less often than this.

New to skin brushing? If you are skin brushing for the first time, start off with a flannel or loofah mitt (used wet) and progress to a skin brush after a few weeks. Don't brush where the skin is broken.

The Value of Essential Oils

When you're detoxing, essential oils can be healing, comforting and balancing. Geranium is restorative and balancing; juniper is particularly cleansing; rosemary helps oily skin and combines well with juniper; lavender is calming and relaxing but also uplifting; both tea tree and lemon oils are detoxifying. The combinations and uses are myriad. Put a few drops in the bath water or into a base oil massaged into your skin before bathing or showering.

This is my favourite detox massage combination (which also seems to help hormonal imbalances and fluid retention):

> 50 ml base oil (I prefer to use extra virgin olive oil, almond oil or grapeseed oil)
> 5 drops each of geranium, juniper, lavender and rosemary.

For more detailed information on the use of essential oils, sneak off to page 117.

Save Us from Cellulite

Is it my imagination, or did anyone ever bother about cellulite before bikinis and cutaway swimsuits? While many doctors still pursue the line that there is no such thing as cellulite, it remains an indisputable fact of female life – and affects fatties and skinnies alike. Inaccurately named during the last century, cellulite was once believed (mistakenly) to be a type of inflammatory condition ('cellule' meaning 'of the cell' and 'ite' indicating 'inflammation').

Cellulite is, in fact, fatty 'tissue sludge'. Although there are many theories on how it gets there, there is a fairly general consensus that it's related to the female hormone oestrogen. A likely scenario is that hormonal changes (brought about by puberty, pregnancy, the contraceptive pill or the menopause) encourage fat cells to become interspersed with fluid. The delicate mechanism which would normally push blood and nutrients to the cells and extract wastes from them is disturbed. The fat cells become enlarged and waterlogged, compressing the capillaries. Lymph drainage becomes sluggish, circulation slows down, oxygen and nutrients don't get to where they are needed and carbon dioxide and other wastes get trapped. No surprise, then, that the skin bruises more easily, discolours, thickens and the skin takes on an 'orange peel' appearance. The bumpy goose flesh

Superskin

is often cold to the touch and, although it can appear on any part of the body, it is most common on the hips, thighs, buttocks, upper arms and, occasionally, the abdomen.

Possible Triggers for Cellulite

* Diets high in fats and sugars
* Diets high in salt
* Packaged foods that contain artificial additives
* Yo-yo dieting
* Missed meals
* Hypoglycaemia
* Diuretic drugs
* Food sensitivities
* Excessive sun exposure
* Cigarette smoke
* Lack of exercise

Cellulite is notoriously difficult to budge, but it is impossible to improve matters. Just be persistent and don't expect overnight miracles.

The Cellulite Solution
Get moving! What all cellulited areas of the body have in common is lack of movement. So it makes sense that to reduce cellulite, you must increase circulation. Brisk walking, rebounding and regular massage can all help to get blood and lymph moving again.

EXERCISE
Take a brisk 10-minute walk every day or 20 to 30 minutes two or three times a week.

If the weather is inclement (or it's dark and, perhaps, not safe to venture outside), then make regular use of a rebounder (mini-trampoline), great for detoxifying, shedding dead skin cells and improving blood flow.

100

Ten or fifteen minutes rebounding (you don't need high ceilings or special clothing) is equivalent to half an hour's hard slog on the tarmac, but without jarring the spine.

Treat Yourself
Regular aromatherapy massage is a very effective way of stirring the lymph to life and helping to banish those skin bumps.

Improve Your Posture
Slouching cramps the breathing, which in turn affects the circulation.

De-stress
Stress has a detrimental effect upon hormones, which can increase the storage of fat. So if you're determined to banish the orange peel, get into some serious stress-busting.

Breathe In, Breathe Out
We do this so automatically that we rarely stop to think whether we are doing it effectively. Deep, steady breathing is not only stress-reducing but also terrific for boosting the circulation. Page 179 has more details.

Exfoliate and Stimulate
Regular exfoliation is essential in the crusade against cellulite, so use that skin brush or loofah mitt! Add lavender, lemon and cypress oils (2 drops each) either to the bath water or mix with almond oil as a carrier and massage into the skin before bathing. If possible, shower or splash with tepid water when you emerge from the bath. After your cool rinse, use the same oil mixture and rub into the affected areas.

Diet Makes a Definite Difference

- Cut right back on saturated and hydrogenated fats.
- Avoid sugar and sugary foods.

- Avoid packaged foods, ready meals and take-aways.
- Check labels for salt, artificial colourings, flavourings and sweeteners.
- Increase your intake of fresh fruits vegetables and salads.
- Drink more water.
- Try detoxifying teas such as fennel, fenugreek and sage.
- Drink less tea, coffee and alcohol.
- Avoid cigarette smoke.
- Choose organic produce wherever possible.
- Increase your intake of dietary fibre.
- Eat little and often.
- Follow a regular detox diet.
- Take a regular antioxidant supplement such as Bio-Antioxidant from Pharma Nord, or Solgar Advanced Antioxidant Formula.

IMPROVE YOUR SKIN CARE ROUTINE

There is absolutely no doubt but that massaging the right kind of creams, gels or lotions into the bumpy bits after your shower or bath can go a long way to dispersing the dimples. Keep in mind that, however convincing the packaging or the advertising may be, no externally applied product will have lasting results unless you are looking after other areas such as diet, circulation and exercise. Having said that, there are some sumptuous treatments available that really do seem to help. My favourites include:

- Boots Grapefruit Oil – cheap, cheerful and effective
- Jurlique Body Contouring & Toning Gel
- Felici Cellulite Massage Cream from Bodywise
- Neal's Yard Cellulite Oil
- Blackmores Evening Primrose + Vitamin E Body Lotion

part 3
....

Beauty on the Outside

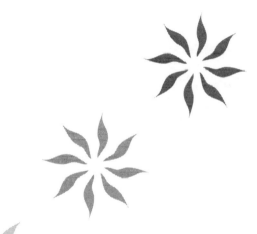

6

Skin Care/Sun Care

As a white candle
In a holy place
So is the beauty
Of an aged face.

JOSEPH CAMPBELL (C. 1881–1944)

Basic skin type is determined by genetic disposition and will usually have become apparent by the age of 12 or 13. But it can also be influenced by a range of other factors too, including diet, environment, stress threshold, how well we digest and absorb our food and the cosmetics and skin-care products we use. Skin condition is affected by illness, fluctuating hormone levels, changes in the weather, lack of exercise, anxiety and trauma and, most times – although not always – by age.

Most people know their skin type, but if you are unsure the following pointers should help.

Dry Skin?

⁕ Flaky patches
⁕ Chaps easily

⁂ Feels tight, especially across the cheeks, forehead and chin
⁂ Prone to itching and irritation

Dryness is exacerbated by exposure to detergents, central heating, air-conditioning systems, smoky, polluted atmospheres, inadequate skin care, poor diet and overexposure to the sun. Check your current cleanser, moisturizer and night cream. Are they right for your skin type or could they be too drying or not moisturizing enough? Given proper attention and the right internal and external care, dry skin can be encouraged to retain more moisture.

Never leave the skin unprotected. After cleansing with a creamy or milky lotion or oil, wipe away any excess with a damp cotton pad, rinse with tepid water, pat dry (use rosewater or orange flower water – more gentle than a regular toner) and, immediately, apply moisturizer. Water itself won't dehydrate the skin, but inadequate rinsing of soap can leave it feeling tight and dry. So rinse really thoroughly. A water splash (repeat it over and over, at least 20 times) helps to improve circulation and encourages the moisturizer, when you apply it after the splash, to be absorbed more efficiently into the skin's surface.

> **In the Know**
> Jojoba and almond oils are not only great for massaging dry skin but are effective make-up removers, too.

Diet-wise for Drys

Drink lots of filtered water.

Increase your intake of cold-pressed salad oils. Use extra virgin olive oil as your main cooking oil for savoury dishes. Snack on sunflower and pumpkin seeds, almonds and Brazil nuts. Eat oily fish regularly and add a daily supplement of Biocare's Mega GLA or Pharma Nord Bio-Glandin.

A Real Treat

Try Jurlique Aromatic Hydrating Concentrate. Expensive to buy but lasts ages. Just 2 or 3 drops in a bowl of warm water morning and evening. Soak a wash cloth and then press the cloth gently but firmly to the face and neck; press and release 10 times. Or cup the water into your hands and splash your face and neck repeatedly. Also available for sensitive skins (see below).

Sensitive Skin?

- Reddens easily
- Subject to broken capillaries
- Aggravated by ordinary soap
- High cheek colour
- Prone to itching and irritation

Ultra-sensitivity is a real nuisance and can apply to any skin type. Reduce adverse reactions by calming and strengthening the skin both from the inside and the outside. Eat plenty of Superskin Foods (see pages 3–35). Add an evening primrose oil or GLA supplement to your diet. A good-quality multivitamin/mineral complex and extra vitamin C are also excellent sensitive-skin supporters. Choose high-quality hypoallergenic skin-care products which are designed especially for your skin type. And check product labels for preservatives, perfumes, propylene glycol and AHAs; all can increase reddening, flaking and irritation to sensitives. And I've found from bitter experience that 'fragrance-free' can still be loaded with additives. If you're trying something new, always ask for samples so that you can test for sensitivity before buying larger sizes.

Instead of an exfoliating scrub – which can increase redness and soreness – use an ordinary facecloth with your cleanser. It removes dead skin cells and impurities just as efficiently as a gritty paste. But remember to change the wash cloth after each use, throwing the soiled one into a hot laundry wash.

Learn to relax. Stress is the worst thing for causing flare-ups.

Diet-wise for Sensitives

As for dry skin, but also:

Avoid spicy foods and alcohol – especially port, sherry, beer and lager. Get tested for food allergies. Some foods, for example tomatoes, strawberries, seafood, food additives and caffeine, can cause irritation.

✿ Oily Skin?

- ✿ Overall shine
- ✿ Visible open pores
- ✿ Coarse texture
- ✿ Tends to 'shed' powder and foundation
- ✿ Prone to spots and blackheads
- ✿ Poor circulation
- ✿ Sallow complexion

Don't be tempted to attack oily skin with astringent lotions. The sebaceous glands will simply overreact by producing more oil. And anyway, toners don't actually close pores and can be heavily laced with irritating alcohol. If you like the freshening feel of a toner, go natural and choose rosewater or orange flower water for dry areas and, for very oily complexions, witch hazel.

For a twice-a-week deep cleanse, use an oil-based cleanser and then rinse with a water splash and wipe excess with a clean dry face cloth. On the days in between, use a cleanser and a lightweight moisture lotion (one designed for oily skin) after cleansing and toning.

Diet-wise for Oilys

Cut right back on saturated and hydrogenated fats. Include extra green vegetables and fresh green salads every day. Drink loads of filtered water. Make lots of fresh juices using cucumber, celery, dark green lettuce, spinach, beansprouts, apples, carrot and raw beetroot.

More help for oily and blemished skins can be found on page 132.

✿ Combination Skin

❋ Oily 'T' zone over forehead, nose, sides of nose and chin
❋ Normal or dry on cheeks
❋ Flakiness to the sides of the nose
❋ Prone to blemishes

As with oily skin, overexposure to harsh treatments can make the oily 'T' panel more active. Use the advice for dry skin and for oily skin to treat these separate areas.

Diet-wise for Combies

Avoid saturated and hydrogenated fats. Use safflower and sesame oil for salad dressings. Cook with extra virgin olive oil. Eat plenty of fresh sunflower seeds and pumpkin seeds. And masses of fresh fruits and vegetables. Avoid sweeteners and sugary foods. Use natural honey instead.

In the Know
Gently does it. Whatever your skin type, it will overreact if you overcleanse, overstimulate, overscrub or overmoisturize.

While it is always sensible to check with your doctor if you have a skin problem, many inflammations and irritations are caused simply by overwashing with the wrong products. Where the diet lacks essential fatty acids the skin is also likely to suffer more from allergic reactions, since there is less natural protection available.

For more advice on special help for different skin types and conditions, see Chapter 8.

✳ Safe in the Sun

Small doses stimulate, moderate doses inhibit, large doses kill.

THE ARNDT-SCHULZ LAW (ESTABLISHED IN 1880)

Only an alien just arrived here from another planet could have missed the message that sun exposure, at best, hastens wrinkling and, at worst, increases the risk of skin cancer. In the UK alone, 44,000 people are diagnosed each year with the disease and 1,500 die of malignant melanoma. Scarier is the statistic that shows the UK to have twice as many deaths per capita from skin cancer as Australia, where a vigorous public information campaign has significantly increased awareness of the dangers and halted the rise in the number of cases.

Wise women have known for centuries that staying in the shade was the best way to keep skin smooth and unwrinkled. Two hundred and fifty years ago it was normal to find that ladies who stayed in the shade showed no signs of ageing until at least 50 years old. It's only in the past half-century that a suntan has become a symbol of health, vitality, sex appeal and status. Prior to that time, sun-beaten faces belonged to the working class who toiled out of doors: the gardener, farm worker or fisherman. Pale skins implied beauty, breeding and upper social class. Then the weather vane veered 180 degrees and sun-worshipping became the fashionable thing to do.

There is no denying that toasting on the beach leathers the skin, hastens the ageing process and increases hugely the risk of skin cancer. Despite dire predictions and advice to cover up and take care in the sun, some people seem to think that crow's feet and life-threatening disease are prices worth paying for that undeniable boost in self-esteem – a tan.

Others heed the warnings literally and are almost afraid to expose even their noses to daylight. But it seems that either extreme could prove to be a health risk.

Completely avoiding the sun can increase the risk of a number of diseases including osteoporosis. That's because of the action of sunlight on the skin is one of the body's major sources of vitamin D, vital for healthy growth, strong bones and teeth. It has also been suggested that sensible (as opposed to excess) exposure may protect us from some *internal* cancers.

Could this be the ultimate Catch-22? Go out and risk one type of disease, stay in and risk another?

Epidemiologists have confirmed that individual genetic make-up – in other words, skin type and how many moles a person has – can be two of the strongest indicators as to skin cancer risk. In addition, pale faces may be more prone to skin cancer than those with olive, brown or black skin. For a few people the risk is there whether they go out in the sun or not. For others, especially those with fairer skin, it is the unprotected and excessive sun exposure that adds so much to the dangers. The most common mistake is to stay pretty much covered up all year and then bare all to the sun's rays on that hot summer holiday.

One thing is for sure: Too much sun makes the skin tough, lined and leathery; well, it's not called 'tanning' for nothing! Baking your bare bits without the protection of moisturizing sun lotions and oils isn't just impetuous, it's plain stupid.

Know Your UVs

The 'A' in UVA is for AGEING. You can't feel UVA radiation.

Ninety-five per cent of the ultraviolet light from the sun is UVA. It's present in ordinary daylight and can get through clouds and through windows. UVA causes irreparable skin damage, reducing elasticity and firmness, encouraging wrinkles and lip-thinning, pigmentation spots and allergies. It alters DNA and increases the risk of skin cancer. A tan won't protect you against it.

The 'B' in UVB is for BURNING. Like UVA it also contributes to DNA damage and the increased risk of skin cancer. UVB radiation will warm and tan your skin, but also causes sunburn. It won't pass through glass or cloudy skies.

Where's the Harm?

Tanning occurs as a direct consequence of damage to DNA, the blueprint that contains the complete code for body construction and repair. Factors in our 20th-century lifestyle, such as exposure to pollution or pesticide residues, not only damage cells and tissues but also use up or destroy the very nutrients we need for protection, preventing or hindering DNA repair. Damage to DNA can then be passed to future generations. If our eating habits are poor and we don't take in sufficient vitamins or minerals to replace those used up, cell mutation could become more likely and repair more difficult.

Extra Protection?

A constant battle rages inside the body between antioxidant defenders and free radicals, those highly reactive molecules which can destroy cells, cause premature ageing and initiate disease. A major area of new research involves the use of antioxidants and, in particular, carotenoids, as an additional guard against DNA damage. Antioxidants, you'll probably remember from the info on page 28, are a collection of vitamins, minerals and enzymes which protect cells from free-radical damage and a degenerative process called lipid peroxidation.

Don't Bake in the Sun – Don't Fade in the Shade

There seems little doubt that short periods of time in the sun are positively beneficial. While mahogany hues are passé, market research polls show that few people are happy to remain pasty and pale. It seems that a tan boosts morale and confidence and makes us feel healthier and more positive. Sensible exposure to ultra-violet light is vital for our well-being. Body rhythms, hormone levels, vitamin D production and calcium absorption are all controlled by the action of daylight picked up by the eyes and transmitted to the pineal gland (situated in the brain in that area of the forehead known as the 'third eye' or seat of the soul).

20 Top Tips for Sun Safety

1. Get outside during all weathers. Fresh air and natural daylight are health essentials.
2. Don't neglect your normal skin-care routine. Keep up with the skin brushing, massage and moisturizing, through summer and winter. Make sure that your daily moisturizer contains UVA as well as UVB filters.
3. Choose sun protection to suit your skin type, and re-apply it throughout the day, especially after swimming or if you've become hot and sweaty.
4. Use a sun block and protective balm on your lips and a very high protection factor on those fast-burn areas such as the nose, neck and tops of the feet.

5   Be careful when buying products abroad; at the time of writing this manuscript, American and European Sun Protection Factors and UVA/UVB ratings were not always the same. And remember that the level of protection will differ depending upon the intensity of the sun and the climate of the country you're in.

6   Don't let the use of sunscreens – or other skin-care products with protective properties – lull you into a false sense of security. Using them doesn't mean it is safe to stay out for long periods of time.

7   Give children maximum protection. Severe sunburn in childhood can trigger melanoma in later life.

8   When the weather warms up, expose skin gradually to the sun. It's the occasional and excessive exposure to hot sun that is believed to be one of the biggest melanoma risks.

9   Go out for a max of 10 minutes a day to begin with and avoid the real danger zones between 11 a.m. and 3.30 p.m. Never ever sunbathe between 12 noon and 2.30 p.m. The sun's rays are strongest and most damaging during this period.

10 Covering up makes sense and is especially important if you have to be out and about in the heat of the day. Go for loose clothing, longer skirts or dresses, trousers and long-sleeve tops. Bear in mind that thin, fine material can still let through UV rays, but also reduces the risk of burning. Don't forget to wear a hat.

11 Remember that tingling and reddening are signs that the skin has had more than enough sun exposure.

12 Never allow yourself to fall asleep in the sun.

13 Be extra vigilant in the sun if you have very fair skin, lots of moles or freckles or a family history of skin cancer.

14 Don't jump in the shower as soon as you get indoors; leave it about an hour. There is some evidence that vitamin D production could be affected if the skin's natural oils are rinsed away too quickly after sun exposure.

15 Take care if sunbathing near to water, snow or ice. The light reflected from them will intensify the effect of UV rays. And

you'll need greater protection the nearer you travel to the equator or the higher you go up a mountain!

16 Eat plenty of antioxidant-rich fresh fruits, salads and vegetables, and drink lots of water – all year through.

17 Take a top-quality supplement which contains antioxidant vitamins C, E, beta carotene and selenium every day. Supplements aren't substitutes for healthy food or for sunscreen protection, but can provide an additional safeguard against free-radical damage.

18 If you are unlucky enough to be affected by sunstroke or heatstroke, get somewhere cool. Rinse or bathe your wrists and forehead in cool water, to reduce your temperature. Drink lots of water and fresh juices, eat extra fresh fruit and take 2 grams of vitamin C every four hours until symptoms subside. Keep Bach Rescue Remedy and homoeopathic Arnica in your first aid box.

19 Another first aid essential is pure aloe vera gel, one of the best soothers for sunburn. Spread it over the sore bits in a thickish layer and allow it to soak into the skin. Also useful as a kind of undercoat before sunscreen goes on. I have tried several brands and found many of them very sticky and uncomfortable to use. My favourite – for its non-stickiness and real effectiveness – is Aloe 99 Gel from Xynergy Health.

20 If your skin is the type that never tans or if photosensitivity prevents you from going out in the sun – but you'd like to have a tan just the same – try a sunless bronzer. They are also useful for colouring the skin before a holiday or special event which demands sleeveless, low cut or skin-revealing clothing. Technological advances mean that these useful artificial tanning creams have lost their ersatz orange pigment and their ominous odour. These days, no one will guess the difference.

In the Know

If you suffer from a rash as a result of being out in the sun, try changing your sun lotion before you blame the sun itself. Some products, even if labelled 'hypoallergenic', have been known to cause this painful and unpleasant reaction. So, too, can some prescribed and over-the-counter medicines. Boils, blisters and rashes and chloasma (localized darkening of the skin on the forehead, cheeks and temples) can all result from the reaction between sun exposure and residues of antibiotics, anti-inflammatory medicines, diuretics, tranquillizers or hormone therapy. Drugs taken within the previous two years can still cause a flare-up!

Author's note: My grateful thanks to L'Oréal and Vichy for their help with research on photo-ageing and sun safety.

7

Essential Oils

Using natural skincare is as logical as eating good, natural food ... Skin-care products are essentially food and nourishment for the skin, so why not treat the skin, our largest organ, with the same care as we do the inside of our bodies? The younger we begin feeding our skin a healthy diet, the younger we will look and stay. And, most importantly, the more we will delay the visible signs of ageing.

DR JURGEN KLEIN, NATUROPATH AND BIOCHEMIST, JURLIQUE

On page 31 I've chatted about how beneficial for your skin it can be to include the right kind of cold-pressed edible oils, such as olive, safflower and pumpkin seed oils, in your diet. Rich in *essential fatty acids*, these natural polyunsaturated oils are, indeed, an *essential* part of a healthy diet. But it wasn't until someone asked me the question at a talk I was giving the other day on skin health that I realized how easy it could be for someone to confuse the *essential fatty acids* found in the oils that we eat with the *essential oils* of aromatherapy. After all, they are both referred to as 'essential' and both are helpful and healthful for the skin.

Buzzword

Aromatherapy is a healing art which utilizes the potent volatile essential oils of herbs and flowers to bring about changes in the body and mind. As esoteric as it may sound, it has a solid scientific basis. Herbs and other botanicals have been used in their whole and natural form through centuries of therapeutic healing. Today, extracts from these same raw materials form a large percentage of the modern pharmacopoeia – drugs available on prescription.

Essential oils are probably best known for their ability to promote physical and psychological well-being, the right blends of oils having the potential to lift us up, wind us down, improve our concentration or calm an overactive mind. But pure essential oils have an extremely wide range of therapeutic properties, including helping us to look after our skins. For example, their normalizing, balancing qualities make them valuable in the treatment of both dry and oily skin conditions and other common skin disorders. They can enhance the healing process following injury, inflammation and infection, as well as encouraging lymph drainage and other important eliminative processes.

In the Know

Essential oils can be found in any part of the plant including flowers, fruit, grasses, leaves, peel, roots, resins, seeds, stems, twigs or bark, and are so-called because they are produced from the distilled *essence* of the plant.

Essentials oils can be:

Anti-bacterial	Cleansing	Invigorating
Anti-inflammatory	Comforting	Pain-relieving
Antiseptic	Confidence-boosting	Protecting
Anti-depressant	Decongesting	Relaxing
Anti-fungal	Deodorizing	Sedating
Anti-spasmodic	De-stressing	Sensual

Anti-viral   Detoxifying   Skin-conditioning
Astringent   Diuretic   Sleep-inducing
Balancing   Energizing   Soothing
Calming   Immune-boosting   Stimulating
    Uplifting
    Warming

Face Lift

This very simple but wonderful facial massage was recommended to me by a facialist and is one that I use often. It goes like this:

Mix 2 drops each of frankincense and juniper with 5 ml/1 teaspoon of sweet almond oil. With a small amount of the mixture on the pads of the fingers and using firm but gentle pressure, make little circles all over the face. Take care not to over-stimulate. Begin at the forehead and work across the temples, then down the bridge and sides of the nose, across the cheeks, around the mouth and chin. Lift the chin and massage the neck with firm strokes in a downward direction; include the sides of the neck and the décolletage until the oil has been mostly absorbed. Take care not to coat the under-eye area with oil, as this can make the eyes puffy. Instead, just tap gently with the pad of an index finger, from the outer eye to inside the bridge of the nose – and back again. Lie down or sit quietly for 10 minutes, breathing slowly and deeply, and then wipe over the skin with make-up remover pads moistened in warm water. Finally, rub the face and neck gently all over with a clean, dry face cloth.

This massage works just as well for oily skin as it does for dry and, if done regularly, can be a useful way of helping to cleanse and clear blocked pores.

Pure essential oils can make a truly valuable addition to the usual stock of face and body care products we keep in our bathroom cupboard. For example for use in the bath, to add that important daily stroke of body lotion or moisturizer or simply to vaporize in the air around us.

To use this same recipe for a body massage, you'll need to double or treble the quantity of both the essential oils and the carrier. Warm the oil in the hands before applying to the body.

✿ In the Bath

Add 2 drops each of the relevant oils (see list below) to 5 ml of carrier oil or full-fat milk and drizzle the whole mixture into the bath water just before you turn off the taps. Don't be tempted to drop undiluted pure oils into the water. They won't dissolve and could irritate your sensitive bits.

Still trying to wake-up?	Rosemary and grapefruit
Need to clear a stuffy head?	Eucalyptus and lemon
Cleansing clean-up?	Clary sage, geranium and juniper
Bath before bed?	Lavender and chamomile
Bathing together?	Ylang-ylang, neroli and vetivert

Take care when you get in and out of the bath. Oil makes surfaces slippery.

For Sensitive Skin

Natracare has a baby lotion that is wonderful for all skin types and all age groups. It is vegan and made from plant extracts and includes vitamin E, vegetable glycerin and aloe. It's great for sensitive skins, light to apply and perfume-free. Available from health stores and from the Natural Woman website (see Resources chapter).

Green People Body Comfort body lotions are completely organic. Smooth to use and beautifully moisturizing, I love their Aloe Vera & Water Lily just as much as the 'no scent' lotion that contains almond and hemp oil. Check out availability in the Resources chapter.

In the Shower?

Add 1 or 2 drops each of your chosen essential oil to a big dollop of unscented shower gel.

For a Cleansing and Relaxing Hand Soak

Find a large bowl and fill it with warm water. Mix 2 drops each of lemon grass and lavender with 5 ml of almond oil. Massage the mixture well into the hands and nails. Then soak them in the water for 5 minutes before drying the excess on an old towel. This is a great mix for tired feet, too.

Carrier or base oils (see below) are used to dilute the essential oils. These natural vegetable oils contain no added preservatives and have a short shelf-life. If exposed to heat and light they will oxidize and go rancid. So it's best to choose top quality cold-pressed oils in small sizes and to keep them in a cool place. Most independent health stores carry a good range.

Which Carrier to Choose

Apricot kernel oil	Helps to prevent moisture loss. Terrific for inflamed or very sensitive skins, and skin that has aged by over-exposure to the sun.

121

Avocado oil	Rich in vitamins. Delicious for dryness, flakiness and for skin that suffers as a result of central heating or air-conditioning.
Evening primrose oil	Good choice for eczema or psoriasis.
Extra virgin olive oil	Makes for a soothing abdominal massage and a low-cost but extremely effective hot oil hair conditioner.
Grapeseed oil	The one for general use because it is very light and quickly absorbed into the skin. Good if your skin is oily or delicate.
Jojoba oil	Pronounce it ho-ho-ba and use it as a face moisturizer or as a luxurious massage oil. Jojoba has a chemical composition close to that of the skin's own natural sebum and is suitable for all skin types, including dry, sensitive and oily.
Peach kernel oil	A first-class face oil to help improve suppleness and elasticity.
Seje rainforest oil	A warming, earthy massage oil harvested from the branches and the fruit of the jessenia palm by the women of the Amazon.
Sweet almond oil	Light and easily absorbed. My favourite oil for face and neck massage and for the hands. It's superb for treating brittle nails and dry cuticles.
Tibetan apricot kernel oil	Produced by Tibetan herbalists from wild apricot trees using instructions from ancient medical texts. An excellent massage oil with good skin-softening properties.
Wheatgerm oil	An excellent choice for healing scar tissue because it's one of the best sources of vitamin E. However, might not be suitable for anyone with a sensitivity or allergy to wheat.

These carriers all have excellent skin-penetration properties. Mineral oil –
i.e. baby oil – stays on the skin's surface, so is not recommended for use
with essential oils.

> In the Know
> Essential oils are strong and need to be treated with respect. Always
> follow the instructions on the bottle or outer pack and don't be
> tempted to use more than is recommended. Twice the quantity will
> not produce twice the benefit.

How to Look After Your Oils

Proper storage is vital if the beneficial properties of the oil are to be main-
tained. Shelf-life, once opened, is around 18 months. Unopened, the
contents should remain effective for up to three years. Citrus oils such as
lemon, grapefruit and orange are not as stable and have a shorter life of
around six months. Quality oils will always be sold in dark glass bottles
with good screw caps. Store the bottles in a cool, dark place and always
replace the cap as soon as you have taken what you need. If exposed to
light and air the oils will be damaged and will evaporate to nothing. Don't
keep your oils near homoeopathic medications.

Buy small quantities of individual oils or blends and replace them as
necessary. Somewhere on the label should be the words 'Pure Essential
Oil'. The term 'Aromatherapy Oil' on its own does not necessarily mean
that the oils are pure; they may have a pleasant smell but provide little or
nothing in the way of therapeutic properties. There are some reports of
unpleasant skin reactions being caused by impure oils.

Pure quality essential oils are likely to vary in price between one
essence and another, cost being determined by the scarcity of the plant
and the time involved in distillation. Ranges of oils which are all similarly
priced are unlikely to be pure.

🌿 10 Favourite Oils

Frankincense (*Boswellia carterii, Boswellia thurifera*)

Good for soothing emotional distress, calming irrational fears and infusing an aura of protection around you. It also has a fine reputation as a wrinkle-reducer. Add frankincense to your favourite moisturizer, body lotion or body oil; this is a strong oil, so you'll need only 1 or 2 drops per bottle or jar. Frankincense also improves breathing, enhances concentration and has a 'protective' quality which eases the trauma of excessively stressful situations. Use this oil if you are a 'shivery' type who feels the cold at night.

Geranium (*Pelargonium graveolens*)

Geranium is balancing, regulating and uplifting – both at a physical and an emotional level. It's useful as a sedative for anyone who is over-anxious and good for hormonal disorders such as PMS, menopausal disturbance, difficult periods and for relieving fluid retention.

A mild skin tonic and a cleansing, refreshing astringent, geranium's sebum-balancing properties make it good for all skin types, from the excessively dry to the most congested of oily complexions. Try adding it to a massage oil or unperfumed body lotion and stroking it firmly into persistent cellulite. Add 1 or 2 drops to a carrier oil and use for gentle facial massage or shake a similar amount into skin tonic and wipe over the face with a cotton wool pad. Use geranium on your detox days.

Juniper (*Juniperus communis*)

Cleansing and toning, juniper is valuable for a number of different skin problems – including acne and eczema. Emotionally, juniper is the one to choose if you're feeling negative or vulnerable. A good 'detox' oil and cellulite treatment, the cleansing action of juniper makes it a powerful diuretic and excellent liver and kidney tonic, helping to purify the blood. Recommended by aromatherapists for cystitis and fluid retention, but not suitable for anyone with kidney disease.

Lavender (*Lavendula officinalis*)

Probably the most versatile of all the essential oils, Lavender is probably best known as the great unwinder. Soothing for all kinds of emotional imbalance, it is sedating, neutralizing and harmonizing. Choose it if you're stressed, exhausted, feeling down in the dumps or have jumpy nerves. Drip a couple of drops onto a tissue and pop under your pillow to calm an overactive mind and to encourage a better night's sleep. Lavender is also one of the best remedies for a headache and for applying to painful or swollen joints.

An excellent skin rejuvenator, the antiseptic properties of this oil make it ideal for soothing and healing blisters, bites, bruises, minor scalds and sunburn. Also for dermatitis, eczema and psoriasis. Considered a very safe oil, suitable for babies and young children, lavender is one of the few that can be applied neat if necessary. Lavender mixes well with – and enhances the action of – most other oils.

Marjoram (*Origanum marjorana*)

Although not used specifically for skin conditions, I include marjoram in this list because it is such a useful oil in other respects. An anti-spas-modic and so one of the best oils for treating muscular aches and pains, on the emotional side marjoram is comforting and reduces nervousness, irritability and anxiety. Valuable to anyone with pre-menstrual problems, period pains or heavy monthly bleeding.

Neroli (*Citrus aurantium*)

Nurturing for all skin types, especially where there is redness, irritation or dryness, neroli encourages the healthy renewal of cells and improves skin's elasticity. Use it if you have thread veins, scarring or stretch marks. Neroli is also for nerves: it calms an overactive mind, aids sound sleep and helps to settle all kinds of depression and anxiety.

Peppermint (*Mentha x piperita*)

Used most commonly for treating digestive disorders and irritable bowel syndrome, just 1 drop of this strong oil blended into a teaspoon of extra virgin olive oil and massaged into the abdominal area will soothe a gripey tum. Because it's a nerve tonic, peppermint is useful for calming anxiety and for lifting depression, as well as dispersing that awful mental fogging we all suffer every now and then. Peppermint oil in a vaporizer helps clear stuffiness – of the nose and the head – and deters biting insects such as midges and mosquitoes. In a footbath it refreshes and sweetens tired, sticky feet and is often recommended by aromatherapists to treat chilblains.

Caution: I must emphasize that this is a strong oil. Use it sparingly and *never, ever* without diluting it in a carrier oil first. Don't use peppermint at the same time as homoeopathic medicines, as it may counteract their effect.

Tea Tree (*Melaleuca alternifolia*)

The essential oil of the tea tree has a very recognizable medicinal odour. Native to southeastern Australia, the plant extracts have been used for centuries by the Australian Aborigines. Tea tree has exceptionally powerful antibacterial, antiviral and anti-fungal properties being one of the best treatments for thrush, fungal infections of the nails and for athlete's foot. Tea tree oil has so many useful properties that it is, not surprisingly, being dubbed 'the first aid kit in a bottle', useful for cuts, grazes, bruises,

Essential Oils

sprains, burns, stings, spots and pimples, cold sores, verrucae and warts.
It is an immune system-stimulant and may be particularly helpful in glan-
dular fever. One of my favourite brands is Thursday Plantation (page 229
has stockist details).

Manuka is the Maori name given to New Zealand tea tree oil.
Although not so widely available, it has just the same valuable properties
as its Australian relative but can be several times stronger. The smell is
also very different, having a woody, sweetly herbaceous aroma – which I
find I like even better than the comfortingly camphorous pungency of
Aussie tea tree. Manuka oil can be found in good independent health
stores. In case of difficulty, contact the New Zealand Natural Food
Company or for mail order, try Xynergy Health Products (see Resources
chapter for details).

Vetivert (*Vetiveria zizanioides*)

Valuable for mature, irritated or very dry skin, vetivert helps to strengthen
connective tissue and promote healthy cell renewal. Also useful for settling overwrought nerves and for inducing tranquillity, it combines well
with ylang-ylang and patchouli to boost sexual confidence and arousal.

Ylang-Ylang (*Cananga odorata*)

Say 'eelang-eelang'. It means 'flower of flowers'. Soothing, especially for
oily skin types because it helps to balance the production of sebum. Also
known for its balancing effect on heart rhythm and respiration, ylang-
ylang is also sedating for the nervous system. Use it to calm and quieten
following severe trauma or shock and to cool anger. Ylang-ylang is
confidence-boosting and effective at helping sexual difficulties such as
frigidity and impotence. Use it with patchouli (in a vaporizer and in the
bathwater) if you are planning the night of your dreams! Be sparing, however: too much of this oil can cause a headache.

⚜ Give Yourself a Fabulous Facial Using Kitchen Cupboard Stores and Essential Oils

Nature's larder has been providing women with organic, additive-free skin care for thousands of years. Be your own beauty counter and treat your skin to a naturally nourishing and revitalizing facial.

Cleanse
Add 1 drop of essential oil of rosemary and 1 drop of lavender to 1 teaspoon of almond oil and massage into your skin to remove dirt, bacteria and make-up. Rinse with warm (not hot) water. Wipe away excess water and oil with a clean, dry face cloth.

Facial Steam
A facial steam helps to release impurities. Fill a large bowl with just-boiled water and add 2 drops of juniper and 2 drops of tea tree oil. Drape a towel over your head to keep in the steam and hold your face over the bowl for 5 minutes.

Gentle Scrub
Exfoliate to remove dead skin cells and unclog pores. Use one of the following combinations:

Oily and combination skins	1 teaspoon oat bran, 1 teaspoon honey, 1 drop lavender oil
Acne	1 teaspoon corn meal, 1 teaspoon honey, 1 drop tea tree oil
Dry, sensitive or mature skin	1 teaspoon ground almonds, 1 teaspoon oat bran, 1 teaspoon jojoba oil

Massage the paste gently into your skin for a few minutes, then rinse with warm water.

Facial Mask

Prepare a facial mask with one of the following combinations:

Oily skin or acne	1 tablespoon of clay (from health food shops), $1/2$ teaspoon honey, 1 drop tea tree oil. Alternatively, blend spinach leaves with watercress and plain yoghurt for a deliciously messy but nourishing and normalizing mask.
Dry skin	1 tablespoon oat bran, $1/2$ teaspoon honey. Or try honey with an egg, 1 teaspoon sesame oil and 1 teaspoon of yoghurt whizzed in a blender.
Mature skin	Avocado, honey and sour cream, or mashed banana mixed with beaten egg.
Sensitive skin	Plain yoghurt, egg yolk and sesame oil.
Combination skin	Mashed strawberries mixed with whole egg.

Apply the mask to the face and neck, taking care to avoid the eye area. Cover the eyes with used chamomile tea bags which have been squeezed and cooled. Lie down, with your feet slightly higher than your head, and relax for a quarter of an hour, perhaps listening to soothing music. Then rinse off the mask with warm water and gently pat dry.

Tone

Make a moisturizing freshener for dry skin by mixing 5 drops of jojoba and 1 drop of lavender oil with 230 ml (8 fl oz) of distilled water. Shake before every use. Soak a cotton ball and smooth over your face and neck. Oily and combination skins freshen up with witch hazel.

Moisturize

Oily skins shouldn't need any more moisture, but dry skins can benefit from smoothing a few drops of warmed almond oil into the face and neck.

Sensitive Skin	Chamomile, neroli and rose oils are good if your skin is temperamental. Add 2 drops of each oil to 10 ml of carrier oil.
Spots and Pimples	Lavender, geranium, neroli and German chamomile added to a jojoba carrier can help to reduce flare-ups and inflammation.
Dry Skin	Instead of lashings of moisturizer that never seem to go anywhere, opt for oils such as geranium, lavender and sandalwood, which help to cure the problem from within – by balancing the skin's sebum production.
Oily Skin	Try bergamot, cedar and geranium in jojoba oil.
Blemishes or Old Scar Tissue	Use vitamin E-rich wheatgerm as your carrier oil and add lavender, frankincense and neroli.
Stress-buster Blend	Mix up the following: 1 drop of neroli, 1 of clary sage and 1 of lavender into a big dollop of non-perfumed body lotion. Massage into hands, feet, elbows and neck.

Recommended Suppliers of Essential Oils

- Jurlique – available from the Naturopathic Health & Beauty Co.
- Neal's Yard
- Nelson & Russell
- New Zealand Natural Food Company
- Passion For Life Absolute Aromas
- Thursday Plantation
- Tisserand
- Xynergy Health Products
- Gerard House

Need More Info?

Both under £3, these two little books are packed with information on how to use essential oils:

Aromatherapy: A Nurse's Guide for Women by Ann Percival
Aromatherapy – A Guide for Home Use by Christine Westwood
(Amberwood Publishing: 01483 570821)
For more detailed information, including some excellent first aid reme-
dies and over 800 'recipes' for everyday use, *Aromatherapy Blends and
Remedies* by Franzesca Watson (Thorsons) is highly recommended.

Take Care

✓ Never apply oils directly to the skin without first diluting them in
a carrier oil. The two exceptions to this rule are lavender – which
can be dabbed onto minor burns and scalds, as long as the skin is
not broken – and tea tree oil, an excellent antiseptic for bites,
cuts and grazes.
✓ Keep all essential oils away from the eyes.
✓ Never take oils internally!
✓ Don't massage if there is fever or high temperature, varicose
veins, skin inflammation, broken skin or recent fractures.
✓ Treat essential oils as you would medicines and keep containers
well away from inquisitive children and pets!
✓ Don't use frankincense, clary sage or chamomile if you intend to
drive or operate machinery.
✓ Don't use citrus oils if you are going out in the sun.
✓ If you're pregnant or planning a baby, seek professional advice
from a qualified practitioner before using essential oils. Some are
not suitable for use during pregnancy.

! Expert Tip
Always keep lavender and tea tree oils in the first aid cabinet: lavender for burns and to soothe a tired body after a stressful day; tea tree
for cuts, grazes and fungal infections.

8

Acne, Eczema, Psoriasis

Dermatology is the best speciality. The patient never dies – and never gets well.

ANONYMOUS

Acne and Oily Skin

Acne vulgaris is a condition most commonly associated with the teenage years and early twenties. The name sounds just about as disheartening as the condition itself, which causes untold misery to millions of youngsters just at a time in their lives when they are striving to look their best. Interestingly, in 'developed' nations acne is believed to afflict around 75 per cent of all teenagers to a greater or lesser degree, but in underdeveloped countries – where processed foods are unknown and junk diets don't exist – acne is not a problem.

It is this single fact which, for me, makes the commonly held medical view that diet has no effect on acne so surprising. Food choices don't make a difference?

Sorry, but I'm not convinced.

Altering my diet was the single most effective factor in eradicating my acne.

Nor am I persuaded by the official view that lack of exercise 'is not a factor as far as we know' and 'lack of hygiene is not to blame either'.

My experience, as a chronic sufferer of acne, was quite the opposite. I've found that exercise *did* help – perhaps because it improves the circulation and assists detoxification.

And what about the cleanliness thing?

Doesn't it make sense that keeping the skin clean reduces the risk of spreading infection?

So What of Medical Options?

The anti-bacterial agent Benzoyl peroxide dries up the spots but, unfortunately, it comes with side-effects such as soreness, irritation and, for me, eczema-like patches all over my face.

Hydrocortisone creams are sometimes suggested, but can thin and waste the skin with prolonged use.

Oral hormones work to reduce the levels of androgens, but doubts have been raised about whether it is sensible to administer hormones to a young person whose own hormones are already wildly out of balance. It's well known that, while the contraceptive pill can reduce acne in some cases, it is also responsible for causing it in others.

Topical and oral antibiotics may help, but have also have side-effects including bacterial resistance, thrush and diarrhoea. Despite this, they remain central to therapy because, as one dermatologist put it, 'Doctors are used to them and they're cheap.' Ah, now, *there's* a really solid piece of sensible medical thinking.

But this dermatologist did also confirm that persistent doses of antibiotics cause side-effects which include a range of gastrointestinal disorders such as indigestion, constipation, irritable bowel syndrome and candidiasis, as well as persistent and recurring infections.

What Is Acne?

Acne is an inflammatory condition of the sebaceous glands, which explains why spots occur where the glands are busiest: on the face, neck, back and chest. Excess sebum blocks the hair follicles and pores, allowing bacteria to build up and form those familiar spots and blemishes. It's a condition most often associated with puberty, a time when *androgens*, the hormones which control the sebaceous glands, are at peak activity. For the same reason acne is also prevalent pre-menstrually and can affect anyone at any age who is suffering from hormonal imbalance.

Possible Causes?

An excess of the wrong kinds of foods, particularly the wrong kinds of dietary fats, does seem to aggravate the sebaceous glands. The usual teenage diet of chips, burgers, cola, sweets, chocolate and other junk food is an open invitation to skin problems.

Acne Aggravators

- ✗ **Hormonal disruption**
- ✗ **Low intake of fluid**
- ✗ **Diets high in sugar, saturated and hydrogenated fats**
- ✗ **Low or non-existent intake of fresh vegetables**
- ✗ **Lack of dietary fibre**
- ✗ **Constipation**
- ✗ **Touching the face with dirty hands**
- ✗ **Squeezing spots and spreading infection**
- ✗ **Inadequate cleansing**

Spots, Bumps, Pimples

Spots, pimples, whiteheads and those little 'blind' bumps are the result of sebum plugging up hair follicles. Blackheads are not whiteheads 'gone dirty'. Blackheads happen when oxygen attacks and discolours the sebum – just as a slice of apple goes brown or a piece of metal goes rusty when it's exposed to the air.

Buzzword

Comedones. A posh name for blackheads. Beware of the comedo- or comedone-extractor – a small metal tool which draws accumulated waste out of the pore or pimple. My own experience of these gadgets is that they are best left to the expert beautician and are not recommended for personal use. Unless guided gently and with dexterity, they can cause bruising and permanent harm.

In the Know

However tempting it may be, NEVER squeeze blackheads. Apart from the risk of cross-infection, there is a strong likelihood that the pores will be so bruised and damaged that they will be unable to work properly ever again. Even touching the face can increase the number of spots and boils.

Not Just Teenagers

Another type of acne, called *rosacea*, is sometimes called 'adult acne' because it's more likely to plague the 30-somethings and older age groups. Common signs include a flushed, red face, sometimes accompanied by severe dryness and irritation around the chin, cheeks, nose and forehead. Skin is often very sensitive to sudden changes of temperature, to certain foods and to some ingredients in skin care products – in particular, perfumes and alpha hydroxy acids (AHAs). It can also be triggered by hormonal imbalances, hormonal drugs and steroid creams. Sometimes associated – incorrectly – with alcohol abuse, severe flare-ups of rosacea can be triggered by the tiniest intake of alcohol, especially port, sherry and spirits.

Digestion Connection

The most likely cause of acne rosacea seems to be faulty digestion, possibly aggravated by certain suspect foods – particularly coffee, chocolate, oranges, orange juice, spices and alcohol, the latter causing swelling and acute redness of the nose.

Several interesting studies show that acne rosacea sufferers may also have hydrochloric acid and pancreatic enzyme deficiency.

Don't Give Up

There is much that can be done to improve skin condition, reduce scarring and discourage flareups, simply by making healthful dietary changes, using tried-and-tested cleansing techniques and taking sensible supplements. Remember that I was told there was no point hoping for a cure? Yet my skin is now in fabulous condition.

As a first step in the treatment of both types of acne, follow the advice in the 'Good Digestion' section on page 79.

In addition I would strongly suggest a consultation with a practitioner who specializes in nutritional therapy. Although not a view supported by the majority of doctors, a very common condition linked to acne is an overgrowth of the yeast *Candida albicans*. Once candidiasis has been treated, it's often the case that the acne improves or clears up completely. However, treatment requires the professional supervision of a qualified nutritionist or doctor who specializes in anti-candida therapy.

Ammunition for Acne

While you're waiting to see a practitioner, the following tips are worth putting into practice to fight candidiasis:

1   Get into the food-combining habit. A good place to start would be my books *Food Combining in 30 Days* (Thorsons) or *The Complete Book of Food Combining* (Piatkus). Feedback from a number of practitioners who treat candidiasis suggests that this very simple food-combining approach – which I have developed over many years – is a cornerstone to anti-candida treatment.

2 From now on, drink more filtered or bottled water – and make it a new daily habit.

3 Cut all sugar, wheat products, yeast and cow's milk foods from your diet.

4 For the time being, bypass any very ripe fruit. The natural sugars that they contain may aggravate the candida condition.

5 Avoid all saturated fats, hydrogenated spreads and polyunsaturated cooking oils. Use cold-pressed safflower, sunflower or sesame oils for dressings and extra virgin olive oil for cooking. Instead of butter or margarine for spreading, use hummus or mashed avocado pear.

6 Add garlic to your cooking (at least a clove a day) or, if you don't like the taste, introduce a good quality garlic supplement such as Garlic Plus from Biocare or Blackmores Garlix Plus Echinacea. Candida *hates* garlic.

7 Eat fresh plain bio-yoghurt every day. If possible, choose one made from sheep's or goat's milk.

8 Avoid alcohol.

9 Invest in a course of gut-friendly probiotics such as Biocare Bio-Acidophilus or Blackmores Acidophilus & Bifidus. Page 229 has more details.

10 Learn more about the condition by reading the *Practical Guide to Candida* by Jane McWhirter (Green Library), which contains a UK directory of practitioners who specialize in treating candidiasis.

In the Know

Certain foods seem to aggravate inflammation, so, if acne vulgaris or acne rosacea is a problem, here's a list of the most common trouble-makers:

☒ Alcohol
☒ Artificial food colourings
☒ Artificial food preservatives

- ✗ Artificial sweeteners
- ✗ Battery-raised eggs or poultry
- ✗ Bread
- ✗ Chocolate
- ✗ Coffee
- ✗ Cola
- ✗ Cow's milk cheese
- ✗ Cow's milk
- ✗ Deep-fried and fatty foods
- ✗ Hydrogenated spreads
- ✗ Oranges
- ✗ Packaged orange juice
- ✗ Peanuts
- ✗ Processed foods
- ✗ Red meat
- ✗ Salty snacks
- ✗ Spicy foods
- ✗ Sugar
- ✗ Sugary and carbonated drinks
- ✗ Wheat-based cereals

Get Steamed Up

Facial saunas help to loosen the blockages associated with acne vulgaris and bring them to the surface. Steam which contains plant extracts such as chamomile, sage, echinacea and aloe vera can make this process even more effective. Face masks and scrubs should, with regular use, also encourage blackheads to the surface. Kaolin masks are particularly beneficial in treating blackheads and whiteheads (known as *milia*); the chalk in the mask is able to attract and absorb the oil in the blocked pore.

Vitamins and Minerals Can Help

Multiple deficiencies of certain nutrients have been found to be common in acne sufferers, possibly as a result of poor diet, poor digestion and absorption or rapid growth. Frequently lacking are zinc, magnesium, selenium and chromium.

Vitamins B_1 and B_2

Vitamins B_1 and B_2 can be useful in the treatment of acne rosacea, perhaps because they're involved in protein metabolism and in feeding the nerves in the skin.

Not All Supplements Are Beneficial

Some supplements can make matters much worse, especially if they are not well absorbed. For example, both iron and iodine can be helpful in treating acne, yet I have found that some supplements containing ferrous sulphate iron or high levels of iodine (such as kelp tablets) are best avoided.

Large Doses of Multivitamins

These can also aggravate acne in some people; low doses are usually sufficient and, in my experience, more effective. A suitable multivitamin complex – containing the B complex vitamins and vitamins A, C and E – should be adequate. Acne in men has shown some improvement following supplementation with a low dose of selenium (100–200 mcg daily).

Vitamin A (as Retinol)

Vitamin A (as retinol) has also demonstrated exceptional in improving both kinds of acne. Where there is a shortage of vitamin A, boils, blackheads and whiteheads appear to be far more common. Vitamin A helps to speed healing, reduce soreness and regulate cell turnover. However, supplementation of vitamin A should only be undertaken with a practitioner's guidance.

Possible GLA deficiency

The overactivity of the sebaceous glands which pump out excess sebum has been linked to a possible GLA deficiency. Regular supplements of evening primrose oil or Mega GLA can be of great benefit to acne and oily skin sufferers, as these supplements do seem to reduce inflammation and 'settle' those over-stimulated glands.

> **In the Know**
> However much you love it, quit the chocolate. Dermatologists don't believe it, but sufferers agree that chocs means spots.

Healthy Diet for Healing Acne

✓ Any fresh fruit (except oranges and orange juices). Aim for two pieces of fruit every day, between meals or before meals but not with other food.

✓ Fresh vegetables and salads. Include a salad and at least two fresh vegetables every day.

✓ All kinds of pulses including butter beans, red kidney beans and chick peas.

✓ Extra virgin olive oil; for cooking and for salads. Try to get a good tablespoonful every day.

✓ Wholegrains such as rice and rye, but avoid wheat-based products as much as possible.

✓ Plain bio-yoghurt (two or three small tubs each week).

✓ Garlic, onions, leeks and shallots. Use them in salads, stews, soups and casseroles.

✓ Seeds and nuts: sunflower, pumpkin and linseeds, brazils and almonds – but avoid peanuts.

✓ Fresh fish twice weekly.

✓ Filtered or bottled water. **It is** particularly important for acne and oily skin sufferers to drink plenty of fresh, clean fluids, including vegetable juices and diluted fruit juices.

✓ One tablespoon of organic linseeds with a large tumbler of water daily.

Caring for Acne and Oily Skin on the Outside

❋ Use the gentlest of skin-care products. It's often thought that oily or acne-ridden skin is tough but, more often than not, it's very sensitive.

❋ Don't bother with powders and foundations. They just increase the risk of blocked pores.

❋ Do use a medicated camouflage. It can hide redness while it helps to dry up inflamed spots.

❋ Cold water splash: The 'action' of cold water on the skin causes a 'reaction' – attracting warm blood to the capillaries at the skin's surface, increasing circulation, improving the transport of healing nutrients and hastening the removal of waste. For very inflamed skin, try a facial wash made from an infusion of the herb golden seal; good health food shops should have golden seal loose or in tea bags.

❋ Choose a medicated moisturizer suitable for oily or blemished skin, and massage a small amount over the whole of the face and neck.

❋ For both types of acne, Bach Flower Rescue Cream or a good chamomile cream can be very soothing and healing.

❋ Preparations containing tea tree oil can be dabbed onto inflamed and spotty areas. Use a clean cotton bud for each eruption, to prevent cross-infection. Tea tree has natural antibiotic, antiseptic and anti-fungal properties and is also useful as a topical application for boils, cuts and grazes. It sterilizes on contact and can prevent microbial growth for several hours.

Cautions: If you have very sensitive skin, carry out a patch test first. Never take tea tree oil internally.

❋ Back scrub: Oily backs are a common problem for acne sufferers. Use a back brush and mildly medicated body wash to gently exfoliate the skin and improve circulation.

❋ Exfoliating scrubs or peeling creams can be a useful treatment for unclogging facial pores and removing accumulated debris. There are lots of excellent ready-made exfoliants available or you can make your own from kitchen ingredients such as oatbran or seasalt mixed to a 'paste' with water. Take care not to scrub too hard, especially over inflamed areas. Cosmetic sponges or flannel face cloths can also help to remove surface skin cells, but it is vital to use a new sponge or cloth for every application to avoid cross-infection. And do be gentle!

❋ Change hand, face and bath towels daily.

❋ Unless you live in an area of outstanding water quality, consider filtering the water you use to wash your face. I have found that chlorinated and hard water can aggravate acne vulgaris, acne rosacea and dry skin conditions.

❋ I have been impressed with a product called Silicol Skin from Saguna. This gel-type face mask contains silicon, a naturally occurring trace mineral which, research suggests, may be of benefit to acne sufferers. The gel is applied to the affected areas, left for 10 minutes and then rinsed off with water. It helps to clear up spots by absorbing excess oil, dead skin cells and bacteria, and it certainly leaves the skin feeling fresh and smooth. Find stockist information on page 229.

❋ If you're distressed by particularly bad acne and don't seem to be able to find anything that helps, I've heard excellent reports from patients who've consulted practitioners specializing in Traditional Chinese Medicine.

Case History

Marie came for her first consultation in February last year. She was 23 years old and getting married in July. She wanted to have 'one last shot' (because she felt she really had tried everything else) at trying to improve her skin condition before the wedding.

Plagued by chronic acne vulgaris since the age of 13, it still covered her face, upper arms, back and shoulders. She had been given increasing doses of antibiotics and steroids over the previous 10 years, had seen four consultant dermatologists and had tried many creams and lotions. Her GP gave her the contraceptive pill, but this had not helped either.

Sometimes the condition would clear a little, but always returned 'worse than before'. Marie's morale was low, she lacked confidence and was shy and reluctant to go out because she said she looked 'so awful'. School days had been miserable as she had suffered unpleasant teasing.

Marie's other health problems included severe constipation, dull and oily hair, mouth ulcers, brittle nails covered in white flecks and a general lack of energy. When she first came to see me her diet consisted mainly of convenience foods, 'TV' dinners, orange squash, white bread, red meat, coffee, tea, a few cooked vegetables and one or two pieces of fruit per week.

Her new diet included many changes and she began to enjoy a range of different foods including plenty of fresh fruit, a salad every day, oat-meal porridge, oat muesli, live yoghurt, fresh fish, vegetables, herbal teas and plenty of water to drink. She decreased her ordinary tea intake to two cups daily, giving up coffee altogether and drinking diluted apple and grape juice and vegetable juices instead. She also enjoyed organic cider vinegar and molasses mixed with hot boiled water as a warming winter drink.

Marie followed a course of herbal cleansing tablets, GLA and antioxidant vitamins A, C and E with a multi-mineral containing zinc and selenium. Her skin was completely clear in time for the wedding, and has remained so. Her hair and nails are much improved, constipation is no longer a problem, she has not had any further mouth ulcers and her energy levels are, to use her own word, 'amazing'. She is thrilled with the recovery and feels much more confident and happy.

༞ Eczema and Dermatitis

The words 'eczema' and 'dermatitis' tend to be used interchangeably to mean the same thing. In fact, dermatitis is a broad term which means any inflammatory skin disorder, including eczema. Contact dermatitis is caused, as the name suggests, by the skin coming into direct contact with a known or unknown substance, such as household or industrial chemicals or plant materials such as rue, viburnum, euphorbia and primula, which can cause severe skin eruptions and irritation in some people.

When the condition referred to as 'atopic', this means that the reaction (in this case, the skin disorder) is triggered by an allergen, for example a food allergy. Atopy is also a factor in asthma and hay fever. Atopic conditions generally run in families. From mild to severe, there are around 20 different types of eczema.

Apart from creams and lubricants either to control or disguise the condition, most of the doctors I've talked to agree that conventional medicine has little to offer. In my experience and in conversations with other practitioners who have specialized in the holistic treatment of skin disorders, natural therapies tend to have a more enviable track record.

Eczema – and other skin disorders including psoriasis and acne – may be a surface manifestation of a deeper internal disorder, such as a build-up of toxins in the blood, an immune reaction to an allergen, hormonal imbalance or stress. Successful treatment is targeted not at the skin in isolation but at whole-body function. There is certainly no single answer to the treatment of eczema; a number of factors need to be investigated.

In the Know

If both parents have been sufferers, then there is a 50 per cent chance of their children being affected. If only one parent had or has eczema, then the risk reduces to 30 per cent. Eczema may also occur in the children of parents who suffer other allergy-related health problems such as migraine, urticaria, hay fever or asthma. Many children who appear to 'grow out of' eczema may be affected by asthma or hay fever in later life. However, there are cases where no family history can be traced.

No one has yet been able to establish what causes eczema, but strong evidence points to a number of areas:

Food Allergy

Cow's milk, cow's milk cheeses, bread and other foods containing yeast, in particular, are known to inflame some cases of eczema. Other trouble-some foods include eggs, peanuts, seafood and soy.

Gut Flora

Depleted levels of friendly bowel bacteria are known to lower immunity. Supplementing probiotics (*acidophilus*, *bifidus*, etc.) has resulted in increased resistance to infections and reduced blistering, weeping and crusting and has proved especially helpful in infant eczema. I was using probiotics successfully to treat eczema in babies and adults more than 15 years ago. Research published as recently as 2001 confirms that probiotics fed to pregnant mums during the last weeks of pregnancy – or given directly to infants if the mother does not breastfeed – can reduce the incidence of eczema by half, compared to the placebo group.

Formula Feeds and Early Weaning

Bottle-fed babies may be more prone to the condition – in childhood and in later life – than those who are breastfed. Weaning too early may also trigger eczema – along with respiratory problems such as wheezing and inflammation of the mucous membrane in the nose.

Liver Health

Although not clinically proven, some experts see a definite link between skin diseases and liver function. I have certainly found evidence to support this theory in my own practice, especially where patients were also suffering respiratory difficulties such as repeated chest infections or asthma. The use of liver-cleansing herbs produces some remarkable results and the successful herbal treatments of Traditional Chinese Medicine are well documented.

Low Immunity and Poor Resistance to Infection

Where dietary improvements, including vitamins, minerals and essential fatty acids have been introduced, allergic reactions may be lessened and symptoms eased in a number of cases. I've certainly found that low intakes of vitamin A, vitamin E, vitamin C and zinc are common to a number of skin conditions, including eczema. Replacing these nutrients through diet and supplements has relieved symptoms for some sufferers.

Biotin Supplements

The B vitamin biotin may have a role to play in the treatment of eczema. Deficiencies of this nutrient have been found in other skin conditions including cradle cap and seborrhoeic dermatitis. Good sources of biotin include egg yolk, cheese, fish, oats, brown rice, potatoes, green and root vegetables, legumes, lemons and grapefruit and lamb's liver and kidneys. Biotin can also be produced in the gut as long as there is enough beneficial *bifidobacteria*. If gut flora is disturbed, this could lead to biotin deficiency and, consequently, to an increased risk of eczema – another good reason to follow a course of probiotics. Biotin is found with other members of the B group in good quality multivitamin and B Complex supplements. Don't go for the cheapest available and do check product labels for information before you buy. It's a general but useful rule that better quality products usually cost more.

Essential Fatty Acid (EFA) Deficiency

We talked about this on page 58. Although researchers still appear divided on whether or not supplementation is of benefit, experience in practice shows that relatively high doses of EFAs such as evening primrose oil are helpful and worth pursuing. There is some evidence that deficiency may be caused by a missing enzyme (delta-6-desaturase, or D6d) needed to convert the linoleic acid from food into usable gamma-linolenic acid (GLA) in the body. I've met many sufferers who say that supplementation of GLA has helped their condition. Evening primrose oil, a well-known source of GLA, is available on prescription for eczema in the UK.

Give hemp seed oil a try, as it is proving increasingly popular and often recommended for the treatment of acne, flaky skin and dandruff, and to help soothe the itching and dryness associated with eczema and psoriasis. But do make sure to choose only organic, unrefined oil. See page 59 for more information.

Herbal Remedy

The herbal remedy *Viola tricolor* (wild pansy) has been shown to have anti-inflammatory and skin-nourishing properties. The beneficial effect is believed to come from *saponins* – soap-like molecules which can soothe inflamed areas – and from the high flavonoid content (see more on the importance of Flavonoids, page 44) which helps to strengthen capillaries. And because saponins can improve blood flow to the kidneys, *Viola tricolor* may enhance elimination of toxins. I've tried this in tincture form (available as Violaforce from Bioforce) and found it useful to take internally and also to apply directly to the skin to reduce inflammation, heat and itching. Page 229 has stockist information.

✳ Psoriasis

Population studies suggest that psoriasis is, essentially, a disease of so-called 'civilization'. It is predominant in the northern hemisphere, affecting over 1 million people in the UK. Conventional treatments range from ultra-violet B treatments, coal tar preparations, skin-softening agents and steroid creams to heavyweight drugs with a heavyweight list of side-effects.

No one knows what causes psoriasis. The characteristic discs of flaky, silvery skin occur when cells reproduce too quickly, sometimes a thousand times faster than normal skin cells. However, some specialists believe that prolonged negative stress, sudden trauma and poor eating habits may all be triggers. It does appear to be the case that deep relaxation techniques, proper rest, fresh air, sensible sun exposure and good nutrition can produce significant improvements.

Sunlight and Fresh Air

Gentle and regular exposure to sunlight appears to speed the healing process. Avoid the hottest times of day; go out in the early morning and later afternoon sun. For protection, take a daily antioxidant supplement and apply aloe gel before and after exposure. My experience with patients has been that sunscreens can aggravate itching and flaking in some people. Another interesting observation is that native Australians who remain in their natural outback habitat do not suffer from psoriasis but can acquire the condition if they move to the city.

Wear Loose, Comfortable Clothing

Check fabric labels. Mohair and wool may be an obvious source of flare-ups. Elastic waistbands, stretch fabrics, polyester and other 'manufactured' fibres don't always allow the skin to breathe, and can increase perspiration and irritation. Clothing labels themselves can be a major source of irritation.

Check Your Laundry

Avoid powders (they don't always dissolve or rinse properly) and choose a liquid wash for your clothes. Steer clear of regular fabric softeners. Go for eco-friendly, phosphate-free products designed especially for sensitive skins.

Another alternative is to change to re-usable detergent-free washing discs, highly recommended for anyone suffering eczema, allergies or dry skin conditions and very economic. They clean all but very soiled items without the use of washing powders or liquids. Eco-balls and Eco-zyme cleaning products are available from Eco-co and The Healthy House. The

Turbo Plus Ceramic Laundry Disc is available from Savant-Health. I use both brands and find them excellent. Further details on page 229.

Oil the Works

Researchers have concluded that the absence of psoriasis in Greenland Eskimos must have something to do with the quantity of fish they eat. I have seen several cases where 2,000 to 3,000 mg daily of Omega 3 fish oil capsules (not to be confused with cod liver oil) made definite improvements in severe psoriasis where low doses made no difference – and also helped a number of cases of eczema, too. For those who cannot tolerate or prefer not to eat fish, it's worth trying nutritional linseed oil capsules in similar amounts. Linseed oil, also called flaxseed, belongs to the same Omega 3 fatty acid pathway as does fish oil. Read more on Superskin nutrients, including those all-important essential fatty acids, on pages 36–66.

Hemp oil can also help. See page 59.

Drink Green Juice

Try adding a daily drink of organic spirulina, wheat grass or green barley to your diet. I have heard good reports from psoriasis and eczema sufferers that these nutrient-rich juices have eased symptoms. I'd go for Hawaiian Pacifica Organic Spirulina from Naturopathic Health & Beauty Co, or Xynergy Health Pure Synergy. Page 229 has stockist details.

Soothe the Surface

Instead of steroid creams, which have plenty of known side-effects, try a natural alternative. The Bach Flower Rescue Cream mentioned earlier is very soothing for irritated, dry and flaking skin. So, too, is calendula cream. Or try Allergenics, a preservative-free, hypo-allergenic emollient cream. All stockist information is on page 229.

Gut Dysbiosis

... sounds horrid but simply refers to a digestive system where the organisms in the gut that usually live amicably together are no longer in harmony. Yeasts and bacteria proliferate and throw friendly flora out of balance. There is some evidence that an overgrowth of the yeast *Candida albicans* may be present in some cases of psoriasis. Removing all sugars, refined starches, alcohol and yeasts from the diet and treating with antifungal medication is a route worth exploring, especially if no other therapies have worked. The book *Beat Candida through Diet* by Gill Jacobs (Vermilion) is a good place to begin dietary improvements. *The Practical Guide to Candida* by Jane McWhirter has more information and a UK directory of practitioners who treat the condition holistically.

Stress

Severe stress, especially that caused by sudden trauma, can be a trigger for psoriasis. Daily deep breathing, regular exercise, massage, reflexology, visualization, meditation, biofeedback and the use of relaxation tapes can all be of benefit, especially when used in conjunction with dietary changes and supplementation.

Colon Cleansing

The American nutrition expert Dr Bernard Jensen has carried out extensive research into a possible link between psoriasis and bowel toxaemia. He has found that auto-intoxication of the blood and tissues, together with a silted and impacted colon, are major factors in skin disease. The cell proliferation associated with psoriasis is increased markedly where unfriendly bacteria have overflowed and penetrated the gut wall. Colonic irrigation associated with cleansing foods and probiotic supplements has shown remarkable results in the treatment of psoriasis. Dr Johnson's book *Tissue Cleansing through Bowel Management* is particularly instructive in this regard – but is definitely not for the squeamish! You'll need a strong stomach to study the colour photographs which show the colonic debris taken from some chronic psoriasis sufferers. For more information on colonic therapy, contact The Colonic International Association (see the Resources chapter and, for further reading tips, the References chapter).

Food Combining

This simple healthy eating system has an excellent track record in helping to reduce the number and severity of allergic reactions in atopic conditions. Improving the way the body digests and absorbs food seems to be especially helpful in eczema and psoriasis. Simple tips such as making sure food is chewed thoroughly before swallowing, sitting down to meals, and resting for a few minutes after the last mouthful are all of value.

9

Hair Care

This is that Lady of Beauty, in whose praise
Thy voice and hand shake still – long known to thee
By flying hair and fluttering hem ...

FROM 'SOUL'S BEAUTY' BY DANTE GABRIEL ROSSETTI (1828–82)

Hair and Scalp Essentials

Hair condition is very sensitive to alterations in atmosphere, environment and lifestyle; any changes in our health and well-being will usually show quickly in the hair. Our 'crowning glory' is not fundamental to survival and so will be the first to lose its supply of nutrients in any crisis. Consequently, hair may appear lacklustre and lifeless, dry and brittle or lank and oily at the earliest sign of stress or illness.

Hair is not just there for decoration or embellishment. It acts to protect the skull and the brain from physical damage, as a screen from the sun's rays, as a valuable sensor (you always notice immediately when someone or something brushes even lightly against your hair) and it keeps the head warm.

The health of the scalp and quality of the hair which grows from it are largely determined by the level of nutrients supplied to the body and how effective the bloodstream is at carrying them to where they are needed. The first step towards super shiny, bouncy, healthy hair is to look after ourselves physically and emotionally. Poor diet and stress can devastate hair health.

In the Know
Each scalp has an average of 100,000 hairs, although blondes usually have more (around 120,000) and redheads fewer (80,000 or so). A natural hair fall in the region of 100 hairs each day is perfectly normal, although shedding will occur in greater or lesser amounts at different times of the year. And if you have ever wondered why hair 'stands on end' when you are nervous or frightened, this is the remains of a reaction designed to make you look taller and terrify your enemy!

Buzzword
Keratin ... is a protein. Each strand of hair is made up of keratin cells constructed in overlapping layers. When the layers lie flat and smooth, each hair reflects the light, making it shine. When the strata are peeling or raised, no light is reflected and hair appears dull and lifeless. Over-exposure to hot sun, drying wind, perming, bleaching, tinting, central heating, curling tongs and blow-drying can damaged the layers of keratin, lifting them and leaving hair looking dry, dull and brittle.

Getting the Balance Right

Hair has its own in-built moisturizer called sebum – the oily substance produced by the sebaceous glands. When hair suffers from dryness, the cause can be often related to lack of sebum production or, alternatively, to the inability of the natural oil to reach all the hair. In long hair or in tight curls, for example, or where hair is damaged, sebum has more difficulty travelling along the hair shaft.

As soon as hair is washed, the sebum coating is lost. But hair left unwashed can create both hygiene and health difficulties; so we overcome the problem by using shampoo and conditioners.

Dull, oily hair may be the result of poor elimination of wastes and toxins, poor circulation, inadequate fluid intake, a sluggish bowel – or of being simply 'below par'. In these circumstances a regular cleansing diet with herbal and vitamin supplements may be called for.

Hair and Hormones

The contraceptive pill, which alters hormone levels in the body, may trigger a thinning of hair in some people. Temporary, sudden hair loss – caused by a reduction in oestrogen levels – can occur in a mother who has just given birth. The hair will grow back, but both of these situations should be helped considerably by the introduction of a multivitamin/mineral supplement and the addition of essential fatty acids to the diet.

Medication

Many medicines – as well as anaesthetics – are known to have a detrimental effect on hair condition, causing hair loss in some people. Also, a sudden whitening of hair can occur following illness or drug therapy. No one should stop taking their prescribed medication without first seeking their doctor's advice, but some dietary changes and well-chosen supplements can make a significant difference to hair and scalp condition in such circumstances.

Condition Is Everything

Whether you are blessed with straight, curly, frizzy, thick or thin hair is determined by your genes. But for those of us who are not satisfied with the type of hair Nature bestowed upon us, it is important to know how to keep treated hair in good condition. Straightening curly hair, perming straight locks into corkscrew kinks, colouring the grey or bleaching in the highlights can all inflict untold damage.

Hair condition can be affected by many other things, too:

Too much sun
Drying wind
Overexposure to salt air
Stress
Chlorinated water
Illness
Nervous disorders
Inadequate rest and relaxation

Lack of exercise
Shallow breathing
Crash dieting
Thyroid insufficiency
X-ray treatment
Chemotherapy
Shock
Trauma

Scalp condition may suffer as a result of:

Seborrhoeic dermatitis
Eczema
Psoriasis

Acne
Dandruff

Hair and scalp can also be detrimentally affected by:

Pollution
Poor-quality diet
Nutrient deficiency

❋ Hair and Scalp Care Plan

❋ Check your diet. Eat fewer of those hair-hinderers and more of the good foods listed on page 160.

❋ Get plenty of fresh air and regular exercise (see page 171).

❋ Sort out your stresses. Excessive negative stress is seriously detrimental to hair health. Page 191 has lots on stress-busting.

❋ Wash hair more frequently. We wash our bodies every day, so why leave hair unwashed for a week? Too long between washes can make for brittle and lifeless hair because dead skin cells and impurities are allowed to build up. Unwashed hair also acquires an unpleasant odour which you may not notice but which can be obvious to others.

❋ Deal with tension. Tightness of the neck and shoulder muscles can affect blood supply circulation – and can be responsible for hair and scalp disorders. Massaging the scalp before every wash will loosen those dead cells, improve circulation and encourage growth. It's good for oily and for dry hair and one of the best stress-busters. Here's how:

Place a thumb behind each ear and spread out the fingers. Press gently on to the scalp and, with the fingertips (not the nails), move the skin of the scalp over the bones of the skull. Work from the base of the back of the neck, upwards and over the top of the head to the brow. Never tear at the hair or rub it vigorously. If you find do-it-yourself massage is difficult, go for a regular professional massage, especially of the scalp, neck and shoulders – and the feet.

❊ Wet the hair thoroughly before shampooing. Use a gentle shampoo and a conditioner at each wash. It isn't necessary to shampoo twice; one application is sufficient. Shampoos that create lots of lather are not necessarily the best kind; the more foam, the harsher the shampoo may be.

❊ Try to use a 'matching set' of products, but don't stick to that same make all the time. Find three or four brands that you like and alternate between them. Choose those which contain vitamins and plant extracts and which haven't been tested on animals.

❊ Rinse hair really thoroughly after shampooing – both before and after applying conditioner. Never use water that is too hot. Warm water is best followed by a cool final rinse.

❊ Don't rub too briskly. Treat hair with extra respect when it is wet. Blot dry and comb through using a wide-toothed comb, GENTLY.

❊ When possible, allow hair to dry naturally.

❊ Every two weeks use a special cleansing shampoo to remove the build-up of gels, mousses and conditioners.

❊ Keep hair-dryer settings low. Damage is not done by drying, but by over-drying and excessive heat, whether from blow-dryers, curling wands or heated rollers.

❊ Once each day brush hair from the nape of the neck towards the forehead and, if possible, bend forwards at the same time so that the blood – literally – rushes to the head. Take care, however; this procedure is helpful to hair but can cause light-headedness. Gentle exercise and – if you are agile enough and do not have heart or blood pressure problems – head and shoulder stands are beneficial.

✳ Don't over-brush the hair. The old wives' tale about 100 strokes per night was recommended in the days before conditioners – to help spread sebum along the hair shaft. But such action can over-stimulate the sebaceous glands, making the hair greasy. Gentle massage is a better bet.

✳ Getting to Grips with Hair Problems

Dry, Brittle, Lacklustre?

If central heating or air-conditioning are getting to your hair, or if you're looking to improve condition, treat with a weekly 'hot oil' pack. For absolute luxury and the most gorgeous aroma, try Jurlique's Hair & Scalp Revitalizer Balm. Or Calendula Shampoo from Neal's Yard. Or make up your own cheap, cheerful and effective alternative by raiding the kitchen cupboard for olive, apricot or almond oil. Add 2 drops of lavender and 2 drops of rosemary essential oils, 4 drops of Bioforce Neem Oil and 1 tablespoon of carrier oil to an eggcup or small bowl and stand the container in a larger dish of hot water. When the oil is warm, massage it gently into the hair. Split open a polythene bag and wrap it over the hair, keeping it in place with a warm towel. Curl up in a cozy corner for 15 to 30 minutes and relax. Then remove the towel and the polythene wrap. Work a good 'dollop' of shampoo into the hair (before wetting it). Then rinse. Shampoo a second time, rinse again, apply your usual conditioner and then give a final and thorough rinse.

Flyaway?

Grapeseed oil is another wonderful conditioner. Two tiny drops rubbed between the palms and then through damp hair works well for all hair types.

Fine?
Shampoo twice and rinse extra thoroughly, but remember that less is more when it comes to most other hair products. Take care not to overload your locks with conditioners, gels, mousses, waxes or sprays; they can all weigh down and flatten your style.

Need to Revitalize?
Pierce open a couple of vitamin E capsules and massage the contents into the roots. Comb gently and leave oil in place for several hours, preferably overnight.

Itchy, Flaky?
If you suffer from seborrhoeic dermatitis, psoriasis of the scalp or dandruff, try the all-natural Gently Medicated Shampoo from Allergenics, Burdock Hair Lotion from Jurlique or the Neem range of hair care products from Bioforce. For stockist details, see the Resources chapter.

Head Lice
These hate Neem oil, too. Try Bioforce Neem Riddance shampoo.

Tired-looking, Dull Hair?
Aloe vera juice is an excellent revitalizer for tired and dull hair. Its chemical composition is very similar to that of keratin, so it is able to penetrate the hair shaft. A few spoonfuls of juice poured over the hair after the final rinse will nourish, protect and add shine. I'd recommend the pure aloe juice from Xynergy Health.

Oily?
Shampoo twice, rinse really thoroughly and use the lightest touch of leave-in conditioner. Avoid regular conditioners; they can be too 'heavy'. Improve your diet (see page 3) and your digestion (see page 79).

Split Ends?

Get your hair cut. Even if you're trying to grow your hair, regular trims are essential. As an emergency remedy and to reduce the risk of split ends, spread a teaspoon of warmed jojoba oil into the ends and leave on for at least half an hour. Try Neal's Yard Coconut & Jojoba Shampoo, which also contains silica-rich horsetail grass, a herb renowned for split ends and good for oily hair, too.

Herbal Hair Rinse

Nettle tea makes an excellent hair rinse and is a useful treatment for dandruff.

Many other herbs are excellent hair-helpers due to their natural anti-bacterial and anti-fungal properties. Chamomile improves hair's shine because it contains natural polymers, which add shine to each strand. Calendula, clove, hops, juniper, rosemary, sage, thyme and yarrow help to control dandruff. Oiliness can be curtailed with wild-cherry bark, red clover or horsetail (which is rich in the trace mineral silica). Horsetail is also believed to be a hair-strengthener, reducing the risk of split ends and breakage. Many of these herbs are now finding their way into hair products.

Trimmings

➡ Keep all combs and brushes scrupulously clean.
➡ Use natural-bristle brushes and wide-toothed combs – they are more gentle on the hair.
➡ Even if you are trying to grow your hair, have the ends trimmed every eight weeks or so.

➡ Always use both shampoo and conditioner after swimming. Simple rinsing without shampoo is not enough to remove either salt or chlorine.

➡ Hairspray landing on the face can cause spots; ask your hairdresser about a plastic face guard to hold in front of your face while spraying.

✿ Good Foods for Hair Health

Live yoghurt, fresh oily fish, fresh vegetables and salads, fresh fruits, cold-pressed oils (but don't cook with them), sunflower seeds, pumpkin seeds, sesame seeds, linseeds, pulses, sea vegetables, wholegrains such as brown rice and oats, buckwheat, millet, almonds, fresh fish, lecithin granules, figs and dates – and plenty of filtered water – are all good for improving the condition of your hair.

Try to Avoid these Hair-hinderers

Too much cow's milk or cheese can be detrimental to hair condition, as can diets high in caffeine, cola, chocolate, sugar, salt, saturated and hydrogenated fats, food additives and nicotine.

Supplements for Healthy Hair

All the B group – particularly B_3, B_5, choline, inositol, para-amino benzoic acid and biotin – are good for the hair and scalp. Find them in all good quality B complex products, such as Blackmores Executive B and Biocare Enzyme-activated B Complex or in multivitamin/minerals, along with important antioxidant nutrients – vitamins A, C, E, selenium and zinc. My favourite multis include Biocare's Adult Multi, Biocare Femforte, Viridian Multivitamin Mineral Formula and Solgar Vegetarian Multiple. Gamma linolenic acid (GLA), fish oil and linseed oil (page 229 has product recommendations) are all beneficial to hair, scalp and skin. And as an add on, I like to take a now-and-again course of Solgar's Sulphur Antioxidant Complex which contains biotin and silica, an important mineral for the health of hair and nails. See pages 60–66 for more information on vitamin and mineral supplements.

Hands and Feet

Nutrition for Nails

If you're fed up with nails that break or split well before they ever reach a decent length, don't give up. A nutritious diet and some seriously good nail care could be all that you need.

When we are run down, going through a difficult or stressful time or recovering from illness, our nails can be one of the first areas to lose strength and shine. In fact, nails – like hair – can be early indicators of health problems long before any other symptoms manifest themselves. The reason is that nails are not considered essential to health and are way down on the list of priorities when it comes to nourishment. But even when we're feeling fine, nails can suffer from exposure to the damaging effects of detergents, hot water, central heating, air-conditioning, cold biting winds and from the continual tap-tapping impact with the keys on a keyboard, typewriter or till.

Fingernails grow slowly, at approximately 1 mm per week. Growth will be slower than this if there is any kind of nutrient deficiency or problem with circulation or general health. And nail growth slows up as we age. On average it takes three to four months for a nail to renew itself from base to tip and about six or seven months to be replenished completely. That's why poor quality nails can reflect a previous state of health as well as a present one.

Caring for your nails really is worth the effort, but be patient; it takes time to achieve results.

In the Know
Nails are the evolutionary remains of claws. In every day circumstances they protect the ends of our fingers from damage as well as enabling us to pick up the smallest of objects.

Cuticle Care

Look after that delicate fold of skin at the base of the nail, the cuticle. It protects the newly formed nail plate, a hard protein made up of live cells which are constantly pushing the nail forward. Once growth reaches the half moon or lunula, the white area above the cuticle, the nail is no longer living tissue – which is why we feel no pain when nail tips are filed, clipped or torn. However, the half moon is still quite sensitive to touch, and care should be taken not to damage or bruise this area when carrying out nail care treatments.

Spotting Signs of Trouble

1   I've seen a number of articles suggesting that white flecks on the nails are a sign of calcium deficiency, but my experience has always been that zinc deficiency is a more likely explanation. One or two marks can simply mean a knock or a bump to the nail, earlier damage to the cuticle or a minuscule air bubble under the surface of the nail. White marks can also be caused by the contraceptive pill.

2   Calcium deficiency is much more likely to be associated with ridged or fragile nails. A lack of magnesium, vitamin A or biotin – a member of the B complex group – or poor digestion and absorption of protein, can also contribute to uneven nails.

3   When nails are curved in a kind of spoon shape or are very pale, iron reserves may be low. If you also have pale skin and are feeling tired, see your GP for a check-up and a blood test for iron levels.

4   Nails that split easily or flake off in layers can mean that the body is lacking essential fatty acids, those vital vitamin-like substances found in nuts, seeds, cold-pressed oils and, in a more concentrated and easily absorbed form, in evening primrose oil and starflower oil supplements.

Super Nail Tips

❋ Fresh lemon juice massaged around cuticles and under nails will lift away ingrained dirt.

❋ Treat your nails to a course of gamma linolenic acid (GLA), the essential fatty acid found in evening primrose oil and other GLA supplements. As a long-term nail improver this is one of the very best. GLA improves circulation (especially helpful to cold hands and feet) and the strength and flexibility of the nail. I have found the most effective dosage to be 3,000 mg of evening primrose oil per day (half that in more concentrated GLA products) for six months, reducing to 1,500 mg daily thereafter. Low doses over short periods of time do not appear to be effective.

❋ A teaspoon of extra virgin olive oil mixed with a teaspoon of sea salt makes a moisturizing nail scrub which helps to soften cuticles and ease away dead skin.

❋ Soothe chewed fingertips, heal hangnails and improve nail strength with Jurlique Nail Oil. I have been testing this for three months and would put it at the top of my list of essential nail products. See Resources chapter for stockist info.

❋ Help to heal cracked cuticles with Nelson's Marigold (calendula) Cream, Jurlique Calendula Cream or Bach Flower Rescue Cream.

❋ Don't forget that any products you use for your hands or your fingernails will be good for your feet, too.

❋ Witch hazel mixed 50:50 with cucumber juice is an excellent remedy for chapped hands. Rub in and leave to dry.

❋ If you're ultra-sensitive to ordinary soaps and detergents, keep a bowl of oatmeal near the tap. It makes a great soap substitute. Wet the skin, rub the hands and nails thoroughly with the oatmeal and rinse with warm water.

Hit that Nail Biting

If you're really keen to kick the nail-biting habit, try these tips:

☑ Ask yourself why you nibble. Stress and worry are major causes. A relaxing herbal remedy such as Kava Kava from Bio-Health, Viridian or Solgar, Valerina Day Time – available from chemists or direct from Biocare – or Bio-Health Chamomile Flowers can help.

☑ You'll be less inclined to bite and chew if nails are short and ⌐-larly filed. And neat, short nails are stronger than long talons.

☑ Treat yourself to a manicure. If you've paid money to have your nails look good, you won't want to destroy the improvements.

☑ It can help to find something else for your hands to do. A friend of mine cured her nail biting by fingering worry beads.

☑ Keep nails – and the skin around them – well moisturized. You're much more likely to attack a rough nail than a smooth one.

☑ Wear cotton gloves in bed and while watching television. Driving gloves can stop that absent-minded nibbling when you're stuck in traffic!

Buzzword
Hangnails are torn areas of skin at the side or base of a nail. They are common where skin is very dry and cuticles are cracked or split.

Nail Care Plan

✓ Always use a barrier cream (my favourite is Natracare Moisturising Barrier Cream) or wear household or gardening gloves for jobs around the home.

✓ Where hands are dry, work-worn or always in water, treat them kindly with Elderflower Hand Softener from Neal's Yard or Jurlique Lavender Hand Cream from the Naturopathic Health & Beauty Company. Always use a hand cream last thing at night. For stressed skin and nails, try Aloe 99 Vitamin E Moisture Balancing Cream. Work the cream thoroughly into the cuticles and very gently push them back as they soften. Doing this carefully every day means that actual cuticle removal is hardly ever necessary. Never trim cuticles with scissors.

✓ Wiggle and stretch your fingers for a few seconds at regular intervals throughout the day to improve circulation and release tension.

✓ Use a fine-grain professional emery board for filing. Never use metal files. File carefully and gently. If nails are very weak, file *before* removing old polish. For toenails, always cut nails straight across, never dig into the sides of the nail. File gently to smooth edges and tidy up. Make trimming easier by using a footbath soak (see page 167 on Feet Treats) before you begin.

✓ Buff the fingernails and toenails once or twice a week. The Body Shop and all good pharmacies sell nail buffers, but a piece of clean rolled-up towelling can be just as effective. Buffing improves circulation and smoothes out ridges, helping to give nails pliability and strength. Buffing also produces a natural polish-free shine.

✓ If you use coloured polish, always apply a base coat to prevent staining and a top coat to help the colour last longer. Clear polish on its own is flattering and makes fingers look longer and slimmer. Don't paint right up to the skin; it can cause nails to soften and stops the skin from breathing. Again, if you use a strengthening polish take care not to paint too close to the cuticle. Tough cuticles are the last thing you need!

✿ Feet Treats

Tips for Toes

Many of the tips I've given you for fingernails work just as well for your tippy toes, too. One of the most ignored areas of body care, it makes just as much sense to look after them as it does to care for your fingernails. Feet work hard for us and deserve extra care. They walk an average of 115,000 miles in a lifetime. They support us and transport us. And yet the 26 bones, 33 joints, 10 nails and the skin which holds them together are usually ignored. Allow neglected toenails to become misshapen and they will probably grow inwards, cutting the skin and causing pressure and pain. In reflexology terms, pressure around the big toe area is often the cause of headaches. We've all used the expression 'My feet are killing me,' and we know how aching feet can make us mega-tired and stressed. So take a step in the right direction and cosset your hard-working feet every day.

One of the quickest and easiest ways to keep feet sweet and in trim is to apply daily hand or body lotion to the toes, toenails, heels and ankles after you bathe or shower or before you get into bed. Skin doesn't get cracked, cuticles don't dry out, nails don't split and the risk of ingrowing nails is reduced. And you moisturize your hands at the same time. Try ALOE Vera and Water Lily Body Comfort Lotion from the Green People Company.

Then, once a week, treat your feet to a massage with apricot or sesame seed oil or peppermint foot cream. Begin with the toes and use a gentle circular massage action over the whole foot including the heels and ankles. It takes only a few minutes to nourish the feet in this way and yet pays huge dividends. It improves circulation, reduces stress and tension, and helps the whole body to relax.

In the same way that we change socks and stockings every day, it makes sense to change our shoes, too. Don't wear the same pair two days together. Choose a sensible heel height. Very flat shoes – and very high heels – can cause posture problems, back ache and spinal misalignment. Help tired feet by taking your shoes off during the day, wiggling your toes and rotating your ankles. Arnica cream helps to relieve the pain of bunions and stiff joints; juniper and lavender oils are also very soothing.

Professional Foot Care

Take yourself off for a professional pedicure. When you see the results, you'll be more inclined to look after your feet.

If you suffer with foot problems of any kind, including ingrowing nails, corns, calluses or fungal infections, see your doctor or ask to be referred to a chiropodist.

Persistent fungal infections can often be diet-related or the result of underlying digestive or bowel problems or an overgrowth of the yeast *Candida albicans*. A consultation with a nutritionist who specializes in the treatment of candidiasis can be a good long-term health investment.

A regular visit to a reflexologist is also highly recommended; this ancient healing art of foot massage can be beneficial for a variety of ailments as well as being extremely relaxing.

part 4
∙∙∙∙∙∙∙∙∙∙∙

Well-being

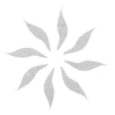

11

Get Moving!

It is not advisable to take violent exercise immediately before nor imme-diately after a meal, as digestion might thereby be retarded.
'ENQUIRE WITHIN' (DAILY EXPRESS PUBLICATIONS, 1934)

The Benefits of Healthy Exercise

I don't need to tell you that regular exercise offers tremendous health benefits. It speeds up the metabolism, burning off unwanted calories and helping us to keep a balanced body weight. It strengthens the heart and the lungs – and the bones – and reduces cholesterol levels. And because exercise can stimulate the production of pain-killing chemicals known as endorphins, it can work to ease pain. It will also give your mood a lift and can boost confidence, too!

Exercise also energizes. However tired you feel, whether you've been standing all day, rushing around everywhere, sitting in the car, working behind a desk or in front of your PC, a change of scene and a change of activity can give the body a real energy boost.

Exercise Is Vital for Skin Health

A major sign of sluggish circulation and toxic overload is a sallow, dull complexion. Because exercise makes us breathe more deeply, improving the circulation and transporting lots of life-giving oxygen and nutrients to all parts of the body, the turnover of old cells for new ones happens more efficiently. Muscles are toned. More of that very important cellular 'glue' called collagen is produced which, in turn, improves firmness and reduces sagging. And because exercise livens up the lymph system, the gut and the bowel, it acts as a kind of internal cleanser, helping our bodies to eliminate wastes and toxins.

Potentially, the greatest bonus of regular aerobic activity is that it helps the body to withstand the bad effects of that most withering of skin enemies – stress.

There are other, more immediate benefits, too: more staying power, boosted energy levels, sounder sleep and mellower mood.

It's got to be worth it!

Please Take It Easy

If you're not given to taking regular exercise, I do hope you'll consider it as an essential part of your day. It doesn't take as much time as you might imagine.

Fifteen to twenty minutes out of every 24 hours?

Half an hour every other day?

Give it a go. But go gently.

Too Tired? Too Busy?

It's all too easy, especially when we are busy or tired, to put it off until tomorrow or dismiss exercise altogether. I know you may not believe it, but once you've found an exercise programme that suits you, you'll find that you really look forward to each session.

'Dos' and 'Don'ts'

Here are a few that I've found really helpful:

Choose Forms of Exercise You Enjoy

If swimming, skipping or stepping don't appeal, you don't own a bike or you think aerobics are boring, go for other options. Learn line dancing or ballroom dancing. Or simply make up your own solo number round the house or the garden.

Rebounding, on a mini-trampoline, is a great way to exercise indoors. Because it's great for the lymph system, it's great for the skin. And 15 minutes on a rebounder is said to be equivalent to half an hour's hard jog, but without jarring the spine.

Don't Stick to One Type of Exercise

Different activities offer different benefits. Aerobic (it simply means 'with oxygen' so you breathe harder) exercise burns calories and fat and strengthens the cardiovascular system and the lungs. Brisk walking, running, cycling, tennis, squash, golf, indoor bikes, treadmills and rowing machines are all aerobic.

Be Flexible

To be good for us exercise doesn't have to be an endurance test. We can also benefit from less strenuous movements which help to improve our strength and flexibility. Simple stretching, lifting weights, dancing, yoga and qi (or chi) gong are good for posture, toning muscle and improving body shape.

Take Care

To reduce the risk of injury, always begin and end any exercise session with deep breathing exercises and warm-up/cool-down stretches. And when you're done, do what the sports stars do. Put on a jacket or top so you don't get chilled.

Make Sure You're Comfortable

Special clothing is hardly ever necessary, but it's good to wear loose, light-weight, breathable clothing and sensible, comfortable shoes.

Go Walkabout

One of the easiest and simplest of exercises is brisk walking. It allows you to ease yourself into a regular activity pattern without overdoing things. And it isn't hard to make it interesting. Plan a new route each day and focus on a destination. Walk to the park or to the local shop. Walk two or three tube stops or bus stops. Go to the post office on foot instead of in the car. Or simply walk round the block. If you're short of time during the day or usually late home from work, you could use your lunch break to walk.

As you move, absorb your surroundings. Notice the architecture or the trees, the plants in people's gardens, the names of the roads and streets. Walking is a great way to learn about your area.

Start Slowly

Whichever activities you choose, don't exercise to extremes. If you're not used to habitual exercise, a 5-minute stint is quite enough to begin with.

Every Little Helps

There are bound to be some days – or weeks – when life is particularly hectic and you just can't commit to the regulation 20 minutes a day. Don't worry about it. Don't feel guilty. But, however tired your feel, don't give up. Exercise is one of the healthiest antidotes to stress and weariness.

Be Diet Wise

Exercise really is as important to a healthy lifestyle as a healthy diet. And healthy eating habits are essential to any exercise programme. So you could say that they're like two sides of the same coin. Although exercise is good for us, it also uses up nutrients which need to be replaced. So be prepared. Just check your cupboard stores and think about your menus for a minute. Ask yourself if you could improve things a bit.

In the Know

A good way of increasing the nutrient levels in your diet is to check your colours. Plan to include not just green but red, yellow, purple and orange foods in your weekly shop. For example, why not eat yellow (grapefruit or banana) at breakfast and add red (apple) to your mid-morning break? Or a bunch of purple (grapes) to that snack? Slice up some orange (bell pepper) to brighten up a stir-fry. Make it a ritual that green (salad) goes great with lunch. Aim to add orange (carrots) and green (beans or broccoli) to your evening meal. Check out the section on Superskin Foods (Chapter 1, page 3) for extra nourishing ideas.

Stay Sharp

Some people might shun walking or running because they're nervous about going out on their own. Attacks are, in fact, extremely rare and it doesn't make sense to let unjustified fear restrict your activities. If you're going out alone, do always let someone know where you're planning to go. Better still, go for a walk or a jog with a friend – it's great fun and you'll help to keep each other motivated.

Face Up to Exercise

Even if we pay proper attention to exercising our bodies, very few of us would ever think of exercising our faces. And yet we all know that improving muscle tone is key to firming the skin. In the struggle against sagging jaws, pouchy eyes and thinning lips, regular facial exercises can truly be face-saving. At the very least they can improve circulation, brighten the complexion and revitalize tired skin.

Unless you are averse to pulling silly faces, you could try *Eva Fraser's Facial Workout*. There is a terrific short version of this in the Sarah Stacey/Jo Fairley *Beauty Bible*.

Alternatively, the *Joseph Corvo Zone Therapy* programme of pressure point massage is more akin to reflexology than massage and an easy system to follow if your life is hectic and you don't have time for a full facial workout.

You may like to try some of the movements from my own Facial Wake-Up which I have enjoyed using for many years. I do these six exercises every day and I'm convinced that they help in many ways. They're especially good for relieving tension, improving circulation and firming the skin and are suitable for trying at home, after your shower or before bed but also fun to do anywhere – in a traffic jam, in the washroom, while you're out for your walk.

Buzzword

We've all heard of *reflexology*, the ancient art of foot therapy which can help to heal other parts of the body. But did you know that the Chinese believe that every part of the body has its own reflex points, including the ears and the face?

Before You Begin

Wash your hands and face, and make sure that nails are clean.

Apply a light moisturizer to the face, but make sure it has been fully absorbed. The skin should feel smooth but not slippery or greasy.

The trick to successful pressure-point massage is to use the fingers or thumbs to move the skin around over the facial bones, not to drag the skin. Work as if you were trying to make 10 little circles over each area before moving along to the next.

It's a good idea to practise first on a table or worktop. Place the tip of your index finger on the surface, press down and then make 10 little circular movements in the same place. Notice how your hand moves around but the fingertip stays put. That's all you need to do for each facial exercise.

1   *Ear squeezing* is a wonderful way to wake up a weary face and a sluggish body and to brighten tired eyes. Gives a tremendous lift if you've been hours in front of a VDU. Work from the lobes to the tops of the ears, using the thumbs and the sides of the index

fingers. First press and squeeze all the way round, then go over the same areas, pulling the ears very gently away from the head. Then, with the pads of the middle fingers, press gently but firmly over all the skin inside the ear crevices. This exercise makes the ears red for a few minutes.

2   *Throat stroking* helps to reduce crêpiness of the neck and improves lymph drainage. Place your fingers at one side of the neck, under the ears, and stretch your hand so that your thumb reaches round to the underside of the other ear. Using each hand alternately, stroke firmly from the chin to the base of the throat. Repeat 10 times.

3   *Forehead massaging* improves concentration and enhances blood flow to the rest of the face. Begin at the centre 'widow's peak' area of the forehead. With the pads of each index finger, press the skin to the skull and work little circles of movement for 10 seconds. Then work your way outwards to the ears and back again until you have covered the whole of the forehead. Pay particular attention to the 'third eye' (between your eyebrows) and to the area above each eyebrow.

4   *Eye-tapping* is said to reduce crow's feet and puffiness but also to improve elimination and stimulate both the large and small colon. Follow the curve of the under-eye and, using the pads of the fingers, simply tap gently from the inside corner, near the nose, to the outer edge and back again. Repeat 10 times.

5   *Nose-pinching:* Light pressure applied to the top of the nose, those little indents where spectacles sit, is said to help activate the kidneys which, in turn, is essential for healthy skin. With a finger and thumb, squeeze and let go over the whole area of the brow bone and sides of the nose.

6   *Cheek-lifting* increases circulation and brings colour to the face. Rest the pads of all the fingers along the cheek bones from the ears to the nose and use them to lift and circle the skin over the bones. Work from the sides of the face towards the nose and

back again, and then down the face to the jaw line, then around the mouth so that you include the areas over the teeth, gums and chin. Pay particular attention to any areas that feel tender. This action is believed to be good for the digestion, helping to improve the way the body absorbs nourishment, and for the lungs, enhancing oxygen supply throughout the body. It's also good for releasing tension in the jaw.

Important

See your dentist regularly. Good dental work, whether it's looking after your own teeth or having proper-fitting dentures, can do wonders for the face and the way it looks. If you suffer from neck, jaw or ear pain, or persistent unexplained headaches, ask your dentist to make sure that your bite is properly aligned. Removable devices such as plastic or clip-on bite adjusters can help not only to relieve pain but may also give the face a firmer image. Work carried out by Dr Nick Mohindra shows that the right kind of dental appliance can improve circulation to the face, reduce lines around the mouth, tighten and strengthen facial muscles and firm the jaw. Wearing a patented and individually-designed dental device called a Facial Rejuvenator for a specified time strengthens facial muscles and, according to Dr Mohindra, significantly reduces signs of ageing. For more information see the Resources chapter.

12

Breathing

Persons desirous of ascertaining the true state of their lungs should draw in as much breath as they conveniently can; they are then to count as far as they are able, in a slow and audible voice, without drawing in more breath. When the lungs are in a sound condition, the time will range as high as from 20 to 35 seconds.

ENQUIRE WITHIN UPON EVERYTHING (1906)

Healthy Breathing for Healthy Skin

When asked for the secret of her longevity (at age 80), the singer and vaudeville star Sophie Tucker replied 'Keep breathing!'

How true! We can survive for considerable periods of time without food, but starve the human body of oxygen and we die almost immediately. Most of us take breathing so much for granted that we can be completely unaware that it is happening; indeed, so ignored is this life-sustaining activity that hardly anyone pays attention to doing it properly. Yet learning to breathe is one of the best ways of channelling nutrients and energy around the body. Strong, deep and full breathing sends life flowing through to the deepest recesses; nourishing, energizing and calming all at the same time.

Breathing is a form of exercise that we could all do with doing more regularly. We really don't do it properly at all. To ancient traditions it is breathing, rather than eating, which sustains the life-force. The oldest known exercise or control of breathing comes from Indian yoga and is called *pranayama*. *Prana* is a Sanskrit word which not only means 'breath' but also refers to the underlying life-force or energy which, the Indians believe, pervades the universe. The *Chi* or *Qi* of Oriental medicine. Hatha yoga, chi (also qi) gong, tai chi, meditation, rebirthing, massage and a host of other therapies recognize the importance of breathing as a healing power for the whole being and, particularly, as a way to mend the mind.

The Chinese concept of health is that developing Chi to its full potential will give abundant soundness, vigour, vitality and longevity. If Chi decreases, body strength and inner energy diminish also. The obstruction of this life-force by poor breathing, inadequate diet, an over-active mind, lack of exercise and mental or emotional distress can result in the body experiencing dis-ease.

To the Western world, unfamiliar with Eastern philosophy, relaxing and resting the physical body doesn't always come easily. In the quietest of rooms and the most peaceful of surroundings, worry wanders in and out of the tranquillity and overactive thoughts seem impossible to eradicate.

A tight throat, clenched jaw, hunched shoulders – even toes gripped claw-like inside shoes – can be so familiar that such mannerisms become part of the person who 'sets' into a rigid, permanently stressed posture. As a result, physical tension is placed upon organs, muscles and bones, particularly the neck, spine and face.

Sadly, many over-stressed people accept their symptoms as a normal part of everyday life and may not even be aware that anything is wrong.

Prolonged and rapid shallow breathing – also known as hyperventilation – means that oxygen and carbon dioxide are exchanged inadequately. This can lead to dizziness, numbness, confusion, poor co-ordination, muscle cramps, chest pain (often mistaken for heart problems), panic attacks and loss of perspective. And, to the great detriment of the skin and all its functions, toxicity! Decreased oxygen supply also increases hormone production from those probably already-exhausted adrenal glands.

Stress blocks the protective prostaglandins which, as well as performing many other jobs, help guard against viral invasion.

Positive stress can be positively good for us. It acts as an incentive, an impetus which fuels our ambitions and motivates us towards further achievements. Spurred on by constructive stimulation, we can feel good and look good, too. Like all emotions, the pleasure and equanimity of our attainments and accomplishments affect our whole being – and show most particularly in the face.

But what about negative stress? When we're under pressure, chances are that our breathing is either very rapid or very shallow, or both.

Glance at the checklist below; if you answer 'yes' to most of these questions, then it may be time to slow down and learn some simple, easy-to-follow deep-breathing techniques. Your skin will certainly benefit.

Do you:

- [X] Always feel tired during the day?
- [X] Find it difficult to concentrate?
- [X] Sigh a lot?
- [X] Feel tightness in the chest?
- [X] Feel that your life moves at an uncontrollably frantic pace?
- [X] Sleep badly or feel unrefreshed after a good night's rest?
- [X] Seethe or suffer from boiling indignation for no apparently good reason?
- [X] Worry about what other people think of you?
- [X] Suffer from otherwise unexplained dizziness?
- [X] Suffer jaw pain or grind your teeth?
- [X] Bite your nails or the skin around them?
- [X] Feel restless when sitting still?
- [X] Experience irregular heartbeats, palpitations, chest pain or tightness not associated with any medical condition?
- [X] Suffer chest pain when anxious?
- [X] Become breathless without exertion?
- [X] Smoke or drink to calm your nerves?

X Suffer from attacks of panic?
X Take tranquillizers for a stress-related condition?
X Bottle up your emotions and find it difficult to express your feelings?
X Cry frequently or feel tearful?
X Feel easily stressed or 'wound up'?

We've talked elsewhere in the book about how damaging stress can be to the health of the skin. The term 'stress' has become the modern idiom for almost any problem related to mental and emotional overload. And I'm sure you've noticed how an overload of negative stress can not only aggravate but also be the cause of physical illness. A study carried out by the now defunct Common Cold Unit (reported in the *New England Journal of Medicine*) found that suffering negative stress nearly doubles the risk of 'catching' a cold. Cancer diagnoses can, all too frequently, be linked to traumatic life events which occurred 12 to 24 months before diagnosis. And no one should be surprised. Where 20th-century pressures, pollution and poor eating habits collide with human animals who have evolved hardly at all since Palaeolithic times, there is bound to be inner conflict.

Skin rashes, urticaria (hives), eczema and psoriasis are often related to dietary difficulties, internal toxicity or a chronic anxiety state, but the medical answer is more likely to be a prescription for drugs or topical creams than a cleansing diet or a relaxation exercise. The patient has already embarked upon the downhill slope towards iatrogenic (doctor-induced) disease because of the negative side-effects, the detrimental interactions of drug cocktails and the reluctance or inability of medical advisers to address the underlying cause of the condition.

Modern-day stress is difficult to avoid. Unlike primitive man we neither run away from nor face head-on the predators Fear and Anxiety which stalk us. Like human pressure-cookers we avoid letting off steam to the point where we are under constant risk of exploding. The effect of this pent-up power puts an unhealthy strain upon all the body's organs. Hormonal glands over-secrete, nerves are 'on edge' and the stomach churns out excess acid. The digestive system shuts down, food is not broken down or absorbed properly and the body is undernourished and cannot repair or renew itself as it once did. High levels of stress are also likely to reduce levels of minerals such as iron, zinc, copper and selenium within the body. Under such circumstances, the skin is bound to suffer.

The Breath Feeds the Body

Deep, sonorous breathing literally feeds the body and the brain. It calms an overactive mind, improves energy levels, reduces fatigue, lessens the risk of chest infections, improves the transport of oxygen and other vital nutrients around the body, enhances the quality of sleep and is particularly beneficial for improving cell turnover and for repairing and conditioning the skin. Correct breathing is a fundamental mechanism for attaining physical, mental, emotional and spiritual well-being. Learning the blessings and benefits of effective and efficient breathing is easy – and free!

In every cell there is a microscopic power-house called a *mitochondrion*, which uses oxygen to burn whatever kind of food that particular cell happens to need, be it glucose, fat or protein.

Poor quality breathing means that the transport of life-giving oxygen (via the bloodstream) to this power-house is reduced. We're not talking about the odd cell or two being affected: there are billions of cells beavering away in your system. They all need oxygen to live. If they don't get fed, neither do you. If they don't live, neither do you.

In the Know

In an area of the brain called the *medulla oblongata* is another gadget known as a respiratory regulator, which organizes the nerve impulses to the apparatus which helps us inhale and exhale. As we breathe in, the intercostal muscles situated between each rib raise the ribcage. The diaphragm moves downwards and the lungs inflate. Because the air pressure inside the lungs is then lower than that outside the body, air rushes in to take up the space. Oxygen is drawn into the body and pushed, again by muscular action, through the bloodstream to the tissues. As we breathe out, the ribs move down, the diaphragm relaxes upwards and the lungs deflate, forcing out carbon dioxide waste and water vapour. This is how your body breathes.

Watch What Happens

Look at the way most people breathe. If you see any movement at all, it's often only the chest which rises and falls. The diaphragm and abdomen hardly move at all. Ask someone to indicate where in the body their lungs are positioned and they will usually point to the upper chest, forgetting – or perhaps, not even realizing – that these substantial breathing bags take up most of the space inside the rib cage. They fill the beehive-shaped area from just below the shoulders all the way down to the curved diaphragm muscle spanning the base of the ribs – and from the spine at the back to the sternum at the front.

The first thing *you* need to do is to find out if you are a belly-breather or a chest-breather.

Put your right hand on your upper chest and the other on your abdomen. Breathe normally, but pay particular attention to the hand which moves the most. If the left hand moves more than the right, you are a belly-breather. If the right hand moves but the left hand doesn't, you could be breathing too shallowly.

Next, place a hand on either side of your ribcage – just as you'd put your hands on your hips, only higher up. Then take a normal breath in – not too deep, just your own average inhalation. Did you feel your ribcage move out sideways? Did the breath push your hands away from your body? If not, you are probably not breathing completely or thoroughly.

If you find it difficult to achieve a deep breathing rhythm, try the following exercise, designed to help you increase your oxygen intake. Don't put any pressure on yourself to 'do it right'; just follow the guidelines and the flow and movement of breath will come. Do the exercise twice a day, first in the morning before you get up to help focus your thoughts for the day, and last thing at night when you're waiting to go to sleep.

Lie down and make sure you are completely comfortable. Be as relaxed as possible. For extra support and easy breathing, you may like to place a pillow or rolled towel behind your neck or knees, or alternatively lie with your knees bent and your feet flat on the floor.

Exhale slowly and completely.

Remember that exhalation is the relaxing part of the breath. Then, inhale freely through the nose. Allow your abdomen to extend and the lower ribs to expand forwards and sideways – but don't be tempted to over-inhale. Breathe to comfortable limits. Do not strain.

Breathe out as slowly as possible, through the nose.

Repeat the in-breaths and the out-breaths 10 times. As you progress you should find that the inhalation will deepen automatically and that the exhalation will lengthen.

If you find yourself taking in only small amounts at each breath, don't be concerned. You may notice that your ribcage and abdominal area move hardly at all. This is a very common experience, especially when you first begin. Regular twice-daily practice will help to increase lung strength and breathing capacity.

During the exercises, keep your mouth gently closed and breathe in and out through your nose. Remember: don't strain. Breathe to comfortable limits.

Exercises to Help You Breathe and Relax

Try them all and then use the ones you enjoy the most.

To Quieten the Mind

1 Lie down in a warm, well-ventilated room.
2 Loosen any tight clothing.
3 Do your basic breathing exercise as usual.
4 Make a picture in your mind of a hamster running around inside a wheel. This is your mind – racing.
5 Watch the hamster for a while. He is running so fast that you can't see clearly the rungs in his circular ladder.
6 Then see the wheel slowing down, slower and slower, until it stops. You can picture the rungs in more detail.
7 The wheel stops going round.
8 The hamster is still there but he has turned over onto his back and is using the wheel as a hammock – rocking gently backwards and forwards.
9 After a while, the wheel stops moving altogether; all is quiet.
10 Finally, picture the hamster getting up out of the wheel and climbing into a huge cozy armchair. In a few moments, watch him fall fast asleep.

The Relaxation Exercise

This simple exercise can be carried out sitting in a straight-backed chair or lying on your back or side. It is said by the Chinese to be helpful for reducing lethargy and tension, stuffiness of the head and chest, and also headaches.

1   Breathe normally and naturally through your nose, with the tip of your tongue touching – gently – the roof of your mouth.
2   Breathe in and out 20 times, counting 'one' for each complete inhale and exhale.
3   Stop counting.
4   Let the tongue relax into its normal position and breathe normally.
5   Then THINK through your body, relaxing each section as you go. Work from the toes and feet upwards, relaxing the legs, buttocks, abdomen, chest, arms, shoulders, neck, jaw, face and head.
6   Return to the feet and start again, this time making sure that the right side of your body is completely relaxed.
7   Then return again to the feet and relax the left side.
8   Lie or sit quietly for 10–15 minutes.

Sitting, Thinking

Sit comfortably, either at your desk, in an armchair, at the dining table, on the floor, even in the car – as long as you're parked up safely.

Close your eyes.

Think through your whole body and make sure that you are as relaxed as you can be. Pay particular attention to those 'clench' traps – the toes, fingers, shoulders and jaw. Breathe normally and with each breath try to slow down both the inhalation and the exhalation.

Progressively deepen the length of each in-breath and out-breath.

On each exhalation say the word 'One' to yourself (like so: W-u-n-n-n-n-n-n-n-n-n-n), either quietly or out loud. Concentrate on this single word; it's a good way of dealing with unwelcome 'mind chatter'.

Each time you lose yourself in this exercise, you should find it easier to relax.

Two-minute Refresher

Relax in a comfortable chair. At your desk, VDU or in your car will do if you don't have an armchair at hand. With the feet placed flat on the floor and slightly apart, allow your arms to flop loosely beside you. Close your eyes, relax your jaw and your shoulders – and breathe deeply. Imagine your arms are made of lead. Let your mind wander for a few minutes. Bring yourself back to reality when you feel ready.

Mental Journey

Picture yourself in a place you've enjoyed visiting: a holiday location, a quiet garden, the majestic grounds of a stately home; in fact, anywhere where you've felt happy and comfortable. Alternatively, retreat to your mental refuge. Close your eyes and imagine yourself in this special place. If you can lie down or sit down, so much the better, but don't worry if you can't. Stay standing, eyes closed, breathing slowly and steadily. Imagine a warm breeze on your face. Let your mind walk around your chosen setting and enjoy the sounds of birds, the rush of the steam train, the waterfall or the stream. See the colours, look at the patterns made by the dappled shade on the tree bark, leaves and flowers around you. When you feel ready, bring yourself back to where you are by taking a deep breath and enjoying a gentle stretch and sigh.

Escape

A variation on the visualization above is to imagine that you're involved in a recreation you really enjoy; it could be cycling, swimming, ski-ing, surfing, rowing or just walking. Don't forget to slow and deepen your breathing. Picture yourself surrounded by beautiful blue water or crisp white snow or a wonderful countryside scene. Perhaps you're cycling down a country lane, for example, or riding the surf. Feel the warmth of the sun and absorb the energy from all the colours and sounds around you. If you're ever physically involved in any of these activities, make a mental note of the sights and sounds which please you so that you can incorporate them into your next visualization.

Face Lift

Tension often shows in the face. Since it takes many more muscles to frown than it does to smile, it's not surprising that grimacing can increase the number of wrinkles. Always remember that cross-patch people get crow's feet but happy people get laughter lines. For this exercise, sit in the same position as above and concentrate on your face. Is your forehead frowning? Are your eye muscles tight? Is your jaw clamped or your teeth clenched? Let the tension go by pulling faces and then relaxing, allowing your jaw to drop. Take in a deep breath, hold for a count of three – one second, two seconds, three seconds – and release the air in a huge sigh. With the out-breath, push away any tension and anger.

Walk the Walk

One of the simplest skin-saving, stress-reducing, mind-relaxing exercises you can do is to go for a short walk. Taking yourself away from the area where the stress and pressure occurred is hugely beneficial. Breathe as you go.

Protect Against Pollution

Breathing in polluted air is an obvious hazard to health. We can't give up breathing, but we can take precautions both to cut down the effects of pollution and to improve the strength and capacity of our lungs.

* If you go jogging, don't do it alongside heavy traffic.
* If you run or walk in a polluted area, invest in a mask. Cyclists wear them; why not pedestrians? The answer may be that people don't find them aesthetically pleasing to the eye. If the designers of high fashion designated protective masks as the latest accessory, our attitude towards them would doubtless change and the shops would run out of stock!
* If you're driving behind a smoky vehicle, temporarily shut off your own vehicle's incoming air. Better to breathe your own carbon dioxide for a few minutes than someone else's carbon monoxide.
* Daily deep breathing exercises indoors or away from polluted areas can help to eliminate accumulated toxins.
* Make sure your diet contains plenty of vitamin C-rich fruits, vegetables and salads.
* Take a 1-gram (1,000-mg) tablet of vitamin C or antioxidant complex containing vitamin C every day.
* Fill your home and your workplace with oxygenating, anti-polluting green plants such as *Chlorophytum* (spider plant), *Spathyphyleon* (peace lily), *Sansiveria* (mother-in-law's tongue), *Aloe variegata* (the partridge aloe) or *Ficus elastica robusta* (rubber plant).

13

Relax, De-stress

A man got onto a bus and found himself sitting next to a youngster who was ... wearing only one shoe.
'You've evidently lost a shoe, son.'
'No, man,' came the reply, 'I found one.'

ANTHONY DE MELLO, *TAKING FLIGHT*

Do Some Serious Stress-busting

Is your skin under stress? When the body and the mind are under pressure, so is the skin. In fact, the condition of your skin can be a very visible register of what is going on inside and underneath that outer surface – so maybe now is the time to take evasive and protective action.

If you're under stress, chances are you'll know it. Or perhaps you don't. The early effects of stress can have a nasty habit of creeping up unnoticed. If your skin has suddenly started to misbehave and you can think of no obvious reason why – no change of water, environment or skin-care routine – then consider that a stressed and overloaded system might be the reason for:

- [X] dark circles around the eyes
- [X] sudden dryness or oiliness
- [X] eczema-like patches

- [x] spots
- [x] blotches
- [x] reddening
- [x] rashes
- [x] dandruff
- [x] cellulite
- [x] change of pallor.

An ashen look is very often a stressed look. Sudden bouts of unexplained itching, sensitivity or a crawling feeling under the skin can be stress-related. If your skin is already on the dry or oily side, stress can simply makes things worse. It can bring on an attack of cellulite – or aggravate the orange peel you already have. Bouts of negative stress, whether emotional, mental or physical – can be the trigger for a long list of other physical symptoms too, including headaches, irritable bowel, body odour, nail-biting and sweating; if prolonged, stress can also be responsible for more serious illness.

Stress is also potentially ageing. Over-production of stress hormones can lead to a slowing down of cellular turnover (or sometimes a speeding up, as in psoriasis), bringing up a backlog of internal 'debris' which can try to escape through the skin. Stress hormones, too, will sometimes be responsible for preventing sleep – and we all know what lack of sleep does to our skin.

Buzzword

Stress isn't caused by the stressful event – the stressor. It manifests from our own individual reaction. Which is why an event or occurrence that is perceived as stressful by one person is so often seen by someone else as nothing to worry about. And vice versa.

✿ Achieving a Balance

Avoiding stress is not the aim here. The right kinds of positive stress are not only enjoyable but good for us. And because everything in life has a balance (every yin its yang), even negative stress can have positive benefits. It's when that negativity becomes overpowering and we lose the ability to recognize the danger signs that the future well-being of mind, body and spirit – and skin – is at risk. The way to deal with things that stress you is to learn to recognize them, see them for what they are, and create techniques to cope.

There are many ways in which we can help the body and the mind to cope more efficiently and less destructively with stress. A good stabilizer for the inevitable stress which nearly all of us suffer is regular relaxation, as much an important part of a healthy lifestyle as nutritious food and refreshing sleep. But relaxation, like regular exercise, is something we usually hear about, promise ourselves we'll get around to – next time the pressure is off – but never do, because we are under too much pressure. Some even dismiss the idea of trying to relieve stress through relaxation because they think it's an impossible goal.

Too busy.

Too stressed.

For some, the ideal way to relax, if they ever get the time, is to chill out on the beach or to curl up with a book. Both these suggestions could bore the Lycra off someone else whose idea of winding down from the daily routine is to get out there and get active. Exercise is, after all, another healthy antidote for a stressful life. It doesn't matter what you choose. Healthy relaxation is about doing something unrelated to work, relationship and domestic pressures. Above all, it should be something you enjoy, something that tips your own stressful see-saw back into balance.

Like any new skill, relaxation is something that takes practice. Giving ourselves, our own personal selves, space can take practice too, especially if we're workaholics or we are trying to cope with more than one job, work long hours and get very tired. When we arrive home completely exhausted, the thought of taking up some other activity is probably the last thing we feel like doing.

More Info?

If you're the kind of person who finds it difficult to give yourself time and space, try this idea. Treat yourself to a copy of *The 10-Minute Miracle* by Gloria Rawson and David Callinan (Thorsons), a fab little pocket book packed full of stress-reducing and revitalizing techniques that take no time at all to do. Carry it with you and refer to it regularly, especially when life is doing its best to beat you. A book I also recommend regularly and have bought for nearly all my girlfriends is *Meditations for Women Who Do Too Much* by Anne Wilson Shaef (HarperCollins), simple daily meditations which really make us think about the pressure we women inflict upon ourselves. The book is designed so you can read one meditation each day, perhaps prior to settling down for sleep or first thing in the morning before the day gets going.

When I suggest that one of the best ways to beat stress is to relax, do I hear you say 'Easier said than done'? Don't forget that when we're relaxed, our minds are less cluttered. The works aren't clogged up with time-wasting 'what ifs', so we are happier. When we're happy, our perspective changes and stressful situations either don't occur or they become easier to deal with.

If you're a stressed, anxious, overworked worrier, here are some of my favourite levellers to help change how you see things. As I once heard a friend's young daughter – aged 7 – exclaim with glee on being asked if she'd been nervous about completing her first water slide: 'I suppose if I'd let it, it could have been scary biscuits, but it was actually a piece of cake.'

Pamper Yourself

Not as a luxurious, occasional treat, but as a regular necessity. To feel comfortable in your own skin, you have to like and to love yourself, to be happy with who you are. In the same way that there will always be areas of our lives that we cannot change, it seems that nobody is ever completely satisfied with the way they look. But instead of dwelling on the bits you'd rather Nature hadn't given you, start to look after all of you. Look after your legs, your feet, your elbows, hands and neck, as well as your face. Appreciate the way your body works for you. Stand tall. Look the world in the eye and be confident that you are a beautiful individual.

Set Aside Some Private Time

Whether it be a few minutes a day or an hour or two each week, be 'off duty' sometimes. Don't answer the telephone. Switch off the mobile. Plan ahead if you like or just go with the flow. Spontaneity can often make an event more enjoyable. Take yourself out for a walk or to a gallery, museum or exhibition you've been longing to see. Or take that book – or that magazine article you thought looked interesting – to a quiet, comfortable spot. Don't defeat the objective by feeling guilty about giving yourself some space. Just do it – regularly – and enjoy the benefits.

Play Joyful Music

– and make room to dance to it. If you honestly can't find time at any other time, then dance around when are doing your chores. Wonderful music really does make light work of making the bed, washing the dishes or cleaning the windows. And music has the power to make you feel better – instantly.

Laugh and Smile Much More Than You Do

Did you know that by putting on a happy face – even if you don't feel like it – your body's cells receive a happy message that is powerful enough to boost your immunity? Laughter and smiles help the body to cope more positively with the effects of stress. Smile right now and you'll see what I mean.

Meditate

There is nothing fanciful or strange about meditation. It may conjure up pictures of Buddha or beds of nails, but to meditate successfully, all you need to succeed is to practise concentration. Picture a colour or a shape that you like, find a pattern in the wallpaper or a tree just beyond the window. Concentrate on it. Every time your mind starts chattering, bring yourself firmly but gently back to your goal. Do this for 5 minutes each day. On the tube, on the bus, at home, in the office – anywhere you like, regular practice quietens and rests the mind and so helps to relax the body and relieve stress.

Take a Walk

A walk can be one of the most invigorating and enjoyable ways to relax and relieve stress. Regular activity helps reduce acidity in the tissues and is a terrific detoxifier. Excessive exercise is as bad as no exercise at all. A short brisk walk every day – or if the weather is awful, a 10–15 minute session on a rower, a mini-trampoline or a stationary bike, or just walking up and down stairs or doing simple aerobics – is enough to improve your mood and your circulation and put back the glow in your skin.

Stay Calm

Don't get angry. It's an unproductive emotion which can upset your immune system, increase the risk of heart disease and age your body.

Count Your Blessings

Like the young man who found the shoe from the quote at the beginning of this chapter, make a note, actual or mental, of the good things in your life: a compliment you've received, a glorious blue sky, finding just the jumper or skirt you were looking for, a lovely meal. See your glass as half-full, not half-empty. Don't be depressed by the weather. See a rainy day for what it is: vital for plant growth, essential for our water supply.

✿ Speedy Solutions to a Stressful Day

✓ **Make a list.** Write down all those things you keep forgetting to do. Take the strain off your brain and give your memory and recall a break.

✓ **Stop and stare** ... into the distance. At something beautiful. Let your mind wander as you watch birds soaring in the sky, listen to water rushing in a stream, smell the wonderful scent of a lavender bush or a jasmine climbing around a cottage door. If you can't be there in reality, wander into your mental picture and lose yourself for a few moments.

✓ **Visit the bathroom.** Freshen your face and hands. Change your shoes. Drink a glass of fresh juice or filtered water. Put on some favourite music. Sit down and chill out for 10 minutes. Then take a walk in the fresh air.

✓ **Treat yourself.** Get off the guilt trip and enjoy the occasional indulgence. Spell the word 'stressed' backwards and what do you get? DESSERTS.

✓ **Keep in touch with friends.** Even if we enjoy our own company, interaction with other people is healthy and vital. Send an e-mail, write a letter. Make new friends by going out and joining in. Make the effort. The world won't come to you.

✓ **Be interested – and interesting.** Don't bore the pants off friends – or family – by never pausing for breath. That's just a quick way to frighten people away. In conversation, remember that the most popular people are those who know when – and how – to listen.

✓ **Don't dwell on problems** that are unlikely to be resolved, or worry about things you can't control.

✓ **Don't try to cope alone.** When a problem that won't go away is making you feel sad and nothing you do seems to help, get help. Talking the problem over with a good friend, a priest (you don't have to belong to a religion or have a regular place of worship), a doctor, counsellor or professional therapist may not produce a tangible solution but can certainly ease the burden and may put things back into perspective.

✓ **Enjoy life's comforts.** Take a relaxing bath in a warm bathroom. Make sure you are not disturbed. Add 3 drops of essential oil of lavender, 2 drops of juniper and 1 drop of grapefruit oil. Relax for 10 minutes. Dry yourself and spoil your body with an all-over moisturizer such as The Sanctuary Body Lotion (from Boots) or Blackmores Body Lotion With Evening Primrose Oil + Vitamin E. Have a freshly washed bathrobe or dressing gown ready to snuggle into.

14

Sleep

❋ The Superskin-saver

A good laugh and a long sleep are the best cures in the doctor's book.
OLD IRISH PROVERB

Getting a good night's sleep sounds simple and yet can be so hard to achieve. Many things interrupt the best-planned slumbers: low blood sugar, nutrient deficiency (particularly of minerals), noise, an unfamiliar room or bed, being too hot or too cold, illness, pain, skin itching and irritation, an overactive mind, excitement, anxiety, worry or depression.

The odd sleepless night can leave you feeling a bit jaded but is unlikely to affect your health detrimentally. Long-term insomnia, on the other hand, can lead to chronic exhaustion – and won't do anything beneficial for your skin, either. Lack of sleep means that your brain is not rested. Fragmented sleep does not give the same value as an uninterrupted seven or eight hours and can lead to irritability, moodiness, poor concentration, an increased risk of accidents and irrational behaviour.

Some people will survive healthily and happily on as few as three, four or five hours per night, their only worry being that they think they should be getting eight hours! But the body is clever and tends to take sleep when it needs it. Research shows that the majority of those who think they get very little sleep are in the Land of Nod for far longer than they imagine.

If you sleep for only a few hours but wake feeling rested, then you shouldn't concern yourself with trying to nap for longer. If you are a '10 hours a night' person that's fine too, as long as you don't wake up befuddled and sluggish.

If you are a long-term and natural insomniac but do not appear to be affected adversely, then settle for the number of hours you do sleep and make productive use of your waking time. If insomnia is something new, try some de-stressing techniques. Stress interferes with sleep more than almost anything else.

- ✓ Invest in a relaxation tape. Use it during the day or play it (on a machine that switches off automatically) while you are waiting to go to sleep.
- ✓ Set aside half an hour each day for rest and relaxation. Make yourself unavailable. The world won't stop turning as a result.
- ✓ Don't eat a heavy meal late at night and avoid stimulants such as coffee, tea, chocolate, salt, sugar, alcohol or nicotine (especially in the evening).
- ✓ Take regular exercise during the day.
- ✓ Buy an oil burner or a vaporizer and some lavender essential oil. Light the burner/vaporizer half an hour before bedtime so that the aroma fills the room. Extinguish the candle or unplug the machine before retiring.
- ✓ Alternatively, put a few drops of lavender oil on a clean tissue and pop it under your pillow. Herb-filled pillows containing plant materials such as lavender and hops are also worth a go.
- ✓ Practise the deep breathing and relaxation exercises detailed on pages 186–189.
- ✓ Soak for 10 minutes in a warm bath and then go straight to bed.
- ✓ Try yoga, tai chi or a meditation technique. Relaxing the mind during the day can mean that you need less sleep at night.

✓ Have regular aromatherapy or reflexology treatments – these help to release tension from the body and aid relaxation.

✓ Learn to catnap – and don't feel guilty about it. Our natural body clocks are designed for two sleeping periods in every 24 hours: one at night and another during the afternoon. Imagine how much less frantic the world would be if everyone went to sleep for an hour or two after lunch.

✓ If a particular worry is keeping you awake, ask yourself if that worry is productive and worthwhile. Usually it isn't.

✓ If you wake up during the night and can't get off to sleep again, don't lie there thrashing about. Read, listen to the radio or a tape – or get up and move around. Record a play from the radio and then listen to it in bed; you should drift off in no time.

✓ If hunger wakes you, it may be that your blood glucose levels have fallen too low. Try a small snack of cereal or yoghurt about an hour before bedtime.

✓ Don't resort to sleeping pills except in extreme circumstances. They are toxic and can be addictive. Short-term use at times of severe distress and anxiety – such as after a bereavement, for example – is entirely justified, but long-term popping of sleep-inducing medication is not recommended.

✓ Try a herbal remedy instead. Bioforce Passiflora drops, Bio-Health Neurotone, Valerina Nighttime, Arkopharma Phytotranq and Solgar Kava Kava all help the body to wind down and relax without the risk of addiction.

✓ A nightly multimineral supplement which includes calcium and magnesium is worth trying for a few months if you're suffering from overactive thoughts, anxiety or tension, especially jaw clenching, restless limbs or muscle spasms. I'd always choose Biocare Mineral Complex, but health stores stock a wide range of products. Just follow my earlier advice and buy the best that you can afford. Cheap products can be a false economy because they may contain ingredients that are not well absorbed.

15

Top Beauty Tips and Products

For stockist information see page 229.

Care for Your Kit

✓ Cleanliness is next to ... Skin brushes, loofahs, flannels and towels. Wash them all regularly – if possible every day. They pick up an enormous amount of dirt and dead skin with each use, and can become happy breeding grounds for bacteria.

✓ Use a jar to wash brushes, rather than a bowl or basin, so that you can keep handles out of the water (wooden handles will spoil and rot if you get them wet).

✓ Never leave brushes to soak: bristles will loosen and fall out. Allow equipment to dry naturally in a warm place, but away from direct heat.

✓ If brushes are stiff when dried, try shaking out excess water more vigorously next time, or rinse them in a drop of diluted hair conditioner.

✓ Before washing brushes and combs, remove any loose hair and then agitate them in warm water and a squeeze of mild shampoo.

✓ Rinse in a basin of cool water swished with a couple of drops of tea tree oil.

✓ Never share your make-up or hair equipment with anyone. If you get an infection such as herpes (see 'First Aid for Skin', page 214), throw your applicators away and start again when the infection has gone.

Look after Your Neck

One of the easiest ways to determine age is by looking at the neck. The skin here has far fewer sebaceous glands than the face, making it more susceptible to dryness and premature ageing. The bust area (the body's natural bra) has no supportive muscle tissue and relies on the elasticity of the skin for support and shape. Test this out for yourself by placing your fingers below your the collar bone and pulling gently upwards. See how the breasts are lifted.

Many women spend several hours a week – and lots of hard-earned money – on caring for the face while ignoring the area between the chin and the bust line. I was always taught that the face ends where the bra begins! In other words, care for your neck and décolletage just as you would your face. Cleanse it, tone it, use your scrub and mask regularly, massage it – and, most important of all, moisturize, moisturize, moisturize! Necks aren't fussy, they're just thirsty.

A five-minute massage with moisturizer at the end of every day really is worth the effort. There are lots of special neck creams on the market, but any good skin cream will do. The important thing is to apply that moisture to cleansed, exfoliated skin and massage it well into the whole neck area, shoulders, back of the neck, up to the ears and over the natural 'brassiere'. With the pads of the fingers, use a circular action, completing each movement with an upwards sweep towards the chin. Do it every day – twice a day if your skin is dry or you work in a drying or polluted atmosphere.

Regular attention will clear away the dry, rough and leathery skin which accumulates at the base of the neck. Caring for this area also improves circulation and lymph drainage and strengthens the muscles which help to prevent sagging cheeks, jowls, jaw and chin. Those with problem skin should find that neck massage improves the blood supply to the face and speeds the healing of blemishes.

Cool water spritzing the face, neck and breasts after applying moisturizer helps to tone muscle and improve circulation and makes the moisturizer twice as effective. On a hot day, a facial spray is super-cooling. At any time of the year, misting can overcome the drying effects of central heating or air-conditioning and provide instant relief for energy-sapping hot flushes. My favourite mists include the plain but simple Evian spray and Neal's Yard Flower Freshener. Or, for sheer luxury, Jurlique Aromamist: try Clarity Blend for that extra energy lift, Tranquillity Blend when you need to slow down.

You can make your own mister using a refillable atomizer, available from chemists and from Neal's Yard Remedies. Mix mineral water with lavender essential oil (35 ml/1 fl oz water to 1 drop of oil) and spray the face regularly throughout the day, blotting the excess away with tissues. Don't forget to close your eyes when spraying and remember to shake the container before each use.

Wrinkle-reducer

Blend 6 drops of frankincense, 3 drops of lavender and 3 drops of neroli essential oil into 100 ml/3 fl oz of almond or olive oil. Massage a small amount very gently into those areas which are already wrinkled or where wrinkles are likely to form. Frankincense is believed to be able to help reduce existing wrinkles; lavender is balancing, calming and helps new cell growth; neroli helps to delay the degeneration of cells and tissues.

Eyes Right

We are blessed with only one pair of eyes, yet we don't always look after them well. These 'mirrors of the soul' are subjected to squinting, bright lights, dust, smoke and make-up as well as plenty of over-enthusiastic rubbing and pulling. Little wonder that some of our first wrinkles appear underneath and at either side of our eyes where the fine, thin skin is particularly fragile.

Eye tissue contains very few oil glands and not that much elasticity, so needs careful feeding. Never be tempted to apply too much heavy cream in the belief that more is better. The skin will soak it up – rather like a sponge full of water, making the eyes puffy and sore. Use products made specifically for the eyes. Apply and remove make-up gently and never rub or stretch the skin.

There are several eye conditions, caused by a variety of factors, which will often respond very favourably to simple dietary changes. For example, there is evidence that cataracts can be aggravated by a diet rich in dairy foods but low in antioxidant vitamins and minerals.

If you have smarting or itching eyes, are sensitive to light or have persistent redness in the whites of the eyes, you may benefit from an increase in wholegrain foods, less red meat, less milk, more fresh fish and more fresh fruit.

If your eye problems have occurred due to diabetes, your diet should be low in animal fats and rich in seeds, nuts, fruits, vegetables and fresh fish. People with diabetes may also be unable to convert beta carotene, the vegetable source of vitamin A, into retinol (essential for eye health). A low-dose supplement of vitamin A in retinol form can be very beneficial in these circumstances.

Puffiness of the eyelids, protruding eyes or heavy bags under the eyes may be symptomatic of thyroid problems. Permanent dark circles can indicate poor digestion and food intolerance. Recurring conjunctivitis can often be related to poor immunity. Dry eyes and a lack of tear fluid suggests a deficiency of essential fatty acids; GLA or evening primrose oil supplements can help here.

Tired eyes will benefit from eye pads made of chamomile tea bags, cucumber slices or cotton pads soaked in herbal Eyebright *Euphrasia*. Extract of angelica is an old herbal remedy used to soothe and repair the sensitive skin around the eye area and is now found in some quality eye creams. Also available as a supplement are Bioforce Euphrasian drops (to be taken orally).

Rest the eyes regularly throughout the day by 'palming': For 2 or 3 minutes at a time, sit in a comfortable chair and rest your elbows on a desk or table. With relaxed shoulders, place your hands over your closed eyes and rock yourself gently backwards and forwards. Breathe deeply. This exercise is especially therapeutic for those working for long hours in front of a keyboard and VDU.

VDU screens

Protect yourself. The air is full of electrically charged atoms. Outside, fresh air consists mostly of beneficial negative ions. Inside buildings, especially those where there is much metal and electrical equipment, negative ions are often in short supply. The highly positive electrical charge which emanates from a VDU screen can change the polarity of the skin from its natural negative state to a positive one. Bacteria and viruses are then more likely to be attracted to the skin's surface, increasing the likelihood of spots, blemishes and, possibly, premature ageing.

Here's how to reduce the risk:

* Take a 10-minute fresh air break every 2 hours. Go outside the building if possible – even on inclement, overcast days.
* Find out if it is possible to open the windows.
* Drink plenty of mineral water throughout the day.
* Don't wear rubber- or plastic-soled shoes while sitting at your VDU.
* Insist on the best quality filter for your screen.
* Invest in an ionizer unit, which helps to increase the negative ions in the atmosphere.
* Take plenty of exercise in the fresh air.
* Take a daily antioxidant supplement.
* Practise deep breathing exercises every day.

❋ Rinse your face regularly throughout the day with fresh clean water, or spray with a water-filled atomizer and then reapply your moisturizer.

Lip Service

The thinnest of skin covers the lips, which is why they are so prone to splitting and even bleeding. Always protect them with a lip moisturizer with a high SPF (see my favourite products page 210); moisture-rich lipstick can also help. Cracks and chaps will benefit from gentle massage with the contents of a vitamin E capsule. Jurlique Lip Care Balm, Bioforce Echinacea Cream or Bioforce 7 Herb Cream and Thursday Plantation Tea Tree Lip Fix are all soothing for lips.

Soap Too Drying?

If you are an enthusiastic soap fan, choose a non-alkaline soap-free cleansing bar or a pH balanced wash-off lotion instead. They may cost a bit more, but are less drying and more kind to your skin. Avoid ordinary tablets of soap, which are alkaline and disturb the skin's natural acid mantle.

Love Those Bubbles?

Bubble bath liquids may be made from strong detergents. If you can't live without the frothy foam, a better option is to add a good dollop of shower gel or moisturizing shampoo to the bath water. Both are less drying than bubble bath or straightforward soap. Do make sure you rinse your skin thoroughly afterwards.

Skin Still Very Dry?

Add a couple of tablespoons of virgin olive oil to the bath water and soak for 10 minutes. Don't use any soap or cleansers. The oil acts as an emulsifier which picks up debris, so you will remove any impurities when you rub yourself dry, but take care, oils make the bath slippery.

Shaving Rash?

Skin brushing – and exfoliating scrubs – are helpful before and after hair removal to prevent in-growing hairs.

Keep some calendula cream in the bathroom cabinet. It makes for a soothing and moisturizing after-shave cream. Widely available from health stores and chemists, my favourites include those by Nelsons and, for sheer luxury, Jurlique.

Skin Redness or Irritation?

Try adding cider vinegar to the bath water (it restores the natural pH), then target particular areas with calendula cream once you are dried off. And get into the habit of applying a general all-over body moisturizer after every bath or shower. It doesn't take long and the benefits really are worth the effort. I love the Neal's Yard Calendula Hand & Body Lotion, also Blackmores Body Lotion with Evening Primrose Oil & Vitamin E. Another favourite is The Sanctuary Covent Garden Body Lotion, which I buy from Boots, but this one does contain perfume. Or I'll add my own essential oils to all-natural, unperfumed lotion. Try Neal's Yard Baseline Lotion or the Natracare Babycare range which comes free of all artificial additives and in recyclable bottles. See page 117 for more on essential oils.

Bath or Shower?

If you have the option, alternate between the bath and the shower. Showers tend to be stimulating (good for bringing you round in the morning), while warm (not hot) baths are best for winding down. Tepid showers are great if you need to be really alert (especially after a late night!), but don't take very cold showers if you have a heart condition or high or low blood pressure.

Stressed or Over-tired?

Make a relaxing potion with an infusion (just as you would make tea) of rosemary and lavender, dried or fresh, and pour it into the bath water. Some shops now sell herbal sachets especially for bath time, but just as useful (and often less expensive) are the herbal tea bags in the kitchen cupboard. Just pop one into the bath while the water is running. It's not a good idea to place fresh or dried herbs directly into the bath, as they can block the plug hole or drain.

Don't soak in the bath for longer than 10 minutes, especially if your skin tends to be dry.

Don't have the bath or shower too hot. This can encourage broken surface veins, may put unnecessary strain on the heart and will destroy the skin's protective acid mantle. It can also contribute to premature skin ageing, for skin cells age more quickly as the temperature of the body rises. Generally when our bodies heat up – for example, during hard physical work – they produce sweat, which not only rids the body of toxins but also cools the blood near the skin surface as it evaporates, then allowing blood from deeper tissues to carry heat out to the surface. But when we are immersed in a hot bath, for example, or even relaxing in a sauna, the body cannot cool itself properly and cellular ageing speeds up.

Make more of your after-bath body lotions, moisturizers and oils. They'll be absorbed more effectively by damp, just-washed skin. Pay particular attention to the knees, elbows, thighs, ankles, heels and hands.

Caution! If you use bath oils, remember that the bath will be much more slippery – so take care!

✿ My Favourites to Encourage Firm and Healthy Skin

Green People Company
Gentle and truly organic formulas for all the family. My top treats are Organic Liquid Soap with Rosemary and Help At Hand cream for dry hands.

Neal's Yard
Of their many terrific products, one of my top favourites is their Frankincense Nourishing Cream. Frankincense is famous for its ability to minimize fine lines. Comes in 40-g and 100-g pots. This is a fabulous revitalizer for mature skins. And I'd never be without Neal's Yard Sun Protection Lip Balm with SPF15 high protection and containing carrot oil. Keep the 7.5-g size in your pocket or bag and the 15-g jar near your make-up mirror. Neal's Yard Baseline Range is fragrance-free and pure, allowing great flexibility and economy for anyone who prefers to add their own base oils, essential oils, flower remedies or infusions to basic products to suit their own personal needs. The range includes bath and shower gels, massage oil, shampoo, conditioner, skin lotion and ointment.

Felici Facial Therapy Cream
I first used this gorgeous moisturizer because I loved the smell (it contains neroli, geranium and cypress essential oils with jojoba), but soon found my skin liked it, too. I use it alternately with the Neal's Yard Frankincense Cream. The Felici product range is available from health stores, some beauty therapists and by mail order from Natural Woman. Felici also have an excellent barrier cream (great for gardeners!). See page 233 for more info.

Calendula Cream
Try Nelson's Calendula Cream or Jurlique Calendula-C Cream for any kind of skin irritation, after-shave rash, abrasions, mild sunburn or insect bites. A good day moisturizer for very sensitive or inflamed skin.

Aloe 99 Gel – Xynergy Health
Non-sticky, well absorbed, ideal for burns and scalds, sunburn, bed sores, blisters and any general skin irritation. I wouldn't choose any other brand.

Blackmores Angelica Eye Nourish
A cooling, soothing gel. Helps reduce puffiness. Great for tired eyes or after a late night.

Blackmores Evening Primrose + Vitamin E Body Lotion
A lovely smooth 'general purpose' body lotion. Economic and delicious to use.

Thursday Plantation
Love their Tea Tree Oil. Superb quality. Anti-fungal, antiseptic, first aid-box essential.

I'd also recommend Thursday Plantation Macadamia Face & Body Oil, superb for dry, sensitive and mature skins. And very economical. Especially soothing for dry legs, arms and feet. Apply sparingly – a little goes a long way.

Samuel Par
Difficult to choose a favourite from this collection of specials for troubled skin. Regular 'dabbing' throughout the day with the La Formule pen should banish painful blemishes. Use it in conjunction with Nightshift.

Also well worth the investment: Samuel Par BodyWash and SkinWash lotions.

Bioforce NeemCare Shampoo and Conditioner
Very effective anti-scurf treatment. Excellent for a dry, flaky scalp. The Neem range also includes a really good riddance treatment for head lice.

Jurlique Neck Serum

Designed to help maintain firm and resilient skin to the neck and décolletage. Pricey, but the most delicious treat for an often neglected part of the body. See more on the importance of looking after your neck on page 203.

Supplements

Flavonoids such as:

* ❋ Solgar's Advanced Proanthocyanidin Complex
* ❋ Viridian Pycnogenol with Grape Seed Extract
* ❋ Biocare ResveratrolPlus High Potency Antioxidant

These flavonoid supplements have potent antioxidant properties which are believed to improve skin condition and elasticity and retard the signs of ageing. Read more about antioxidants on page 28.

Solgar Milk Thistle or Biocare Silymarin Complex	For liver support. Take a one- or two-month course every now and then.
Phytobronz Plus from Arkopharma	Not a sunscreen, but said to provide antioxidant support for anyone who is out in the sun.
Pharma Nord Co-Enzyme Q10	Has major antioxidant properties and is one of the best supplements for improving energy levels.
Biocare Femforte Multivitamin/mineral for women	I've used this supplement for many years and still rate it as the best multi for women.

Blackmores Bio-C

A low-acid vitamin C complex that is kind to the digestion. I take 1 or 2 grams every day and increase to 4 grams daily if I'm travelling in a polluted city area, driving in heavy traffic or think I may be going down with a cold.

Bioforce Echinaforce drops

I would never be without this amazing supplement in my first-aid cupboard. Take with vitamin C at the very first sign of any cold or infection.

Linusit Gold Linseeds

One of the gentlest and most effective of dietary fibres. Why have I listed it under skin care? Because it's such an excellent internal cleanser – so a good skin food, too. Two teaspoons per day with a large tumbler of water is an excellent way to keep the bowels moving and to ease the symptoms of constipation and irritable bowel syndrome. Available from good health stores. Buy only the golden coloured seeds. Avoid brown linseeds and any seeds that are sold loose or are not in airtight packaging.

First Aid for Skin

Quick thinking and the application of first aid can make a huge difference in easing the pain of skin problems, from cracked lips and cold sores to insect bites and burns. First aid can also prevent a worsening of any condition and encourage rapid healing. It needn't be complicated – these treatments can be applied at home, often using ingredients from the kitchen cupboard such as tea bags, vegetable peelings, olive oil and honey. Herbal infusions, homoeopathic remedies and vitamin and mineral supplements also help to promote a speedy but gentle return to skin health. Do remember that these remedies are for first aid only. In the event of a serious injury always seek urgent medical attention.

Bites and Stings

If there is a sting, remove it if possible and seek medical help if necessary.

For wasp stings, pouring cider vinegar over the damaged area helps to draw the poison out, cleanse the wound and reduce the inflammation.

For bee stings, apply bicarbonate of soda solution. And check with your GP as soon as possible; stings can cause unpleasant adverse reactions.

Ant bites can be painful; apply crushed garlic or rub the sore area with cucumber skin.

If you are bitten or stung, take 2 grams of vitamin C (Blackmores, Solgar or Viridian) every three hours and a B complex which contains

25–50 mg each of B$_5$ and B$_6$ (try Blackmores or Biocare): these nutrients all have natural antihistamine properties and are good for distress.

Also recommended are homoeopathic Arnica and Bach Rescue Remedy which may help reduce shock, bruising and swelling.

Add Thursday Plantation Tea Tree Oil or Xynergy Biogenic Aloe juice to cooled boiled water to make an antiseptic wash. Or use Aloe 99 Gel, applied in a thick layer and allowed to dry.

Homoeopathic *Apis mellifica* (Apis mel 30c) is helpful for stings which cause reddening, swelling and pain.

Important caution: Don't take tea tree oil internally or use it for stings inside the mouth.

If you're visiting a mosquito- or midge-ridden area, swallow the equivalent of two fresh cloves of garlic every day, either raw, in cooking or as supplements. Mosquitoes and other biting insects hate the taste and smell and so are more likely to leave you alone.

Neem Insect Repellent from Bioforce is a travel bag essential. Apply it to exposed skin – especially ankles, arms, neck and around the ears – before any outdoor activities and if you are likely to be outside after dark.

If you are attacked by midges or mosquitoes, bathe the bite with a soaked chamomile tea bag or rub with fresh elder leaves and crushed raw garlic.

To relieve the itching caused by a mosquito bite, dissolve 2 teaspoons of baking powder in warm water and bathe the affected area. Alternatively, use a dilute solution of cider vinegar (1 part vinegar to 6 parts water).

Take a B complex (25 mg three times a day) while you are exposed to mosquitoes.

The essential oil citronella is a useful insect repellent, either applied with a carrier oil to the skin or used in an oil burner, especially during the night.

Take artemesia (wormwood) capsules – available from Biocare and from specialist pharmacies such as Neal's Yard and Apotheke – for two weeks before travelling and continue to use during any visit abroad. This herbal medicine is proving beneficial in the treatment of malaria and may also be helpful following mosquito attack.

If you're unlucky enough to pick up a sheep tick (they're common wherever there are livestock or wild animals and in grassland and over-grown scrub), one of the quickest ways to deal with them is to drop neat tea tree oil on to the skin. The tick usually lets go pretty quickly. If you need extra help, grab the tick with a pair of eyebrow tweezers and twist anti-clockwise. Re-apply the tea tree oil throughout the day and for the next few days to reduce the risk of the bite becoming infected.

✿ Brittle, Splitting and Flaking Nails

Massage the contents of a cod liver oil capsule and a vitamin E capsule into the nails every night (wear cotton gloves in bed if the smell or sticki-ness disturbs you) and take GLA or evening primrose oil supplements every day. GLA supplements – such as Pharma Nord Bio-Glandin and Mega GLA from Biocare – are, in my view, among the best nail strength-eners, but do bear in mind that you need to take the full recommended dose for at least 8 weeks before you'll see any improvements. (Also see Chapters 2 and 10.)

✿ Broken Veins

Damage to tiny capillaries occurs most commonly in areas where there is poor circulation and where thinner or ultra-sensitive skin is exposed to the atmosphere. Fragile capillary walls dilate and rupture, allowing blood to seep out into the tissues in minute quantities. The face and legs seem particularly susceptible. High blood pressure (hypertension) and some medicines such as steroids and hydrocortisone creams can aggravate the problem.

Avoid very hot or very cold foods, spices, alcohol, salt, coffee and sugar.

Increase your intake of fresh fruit – especially grapefruit, lemons, apples and avocados – and of raw beetroot, almonds, Brazil nuts, sunflower and pumpkin seeds, sprouted seeds and grains, eggs and cold-pressed oils.

Supplement with a top quality antioxidant such as Biocare's ResveratrolPlus, Viridian Pycnogenol or Solgar Advanced Proanthocyanidin Complex, plus a good quality vitamin C (1,000–2,000 mg daily) and vitamin E (100–400 iu daily).

Protect the skin against the drying effects of cold wind, central heating and air-conditioning by always applying protective moisturizer and spraying the face regularly throughout the day with a water-mist. Some cosmetic companies produce very portable ready-to-use sprays made from mineral water and humectants – or you could refill your own atomizer with filtered or spring water or try one of the spritzers recommended on page 204.

☀ Bumps and Bruises

Unless the skin is broken, rub the area gently but firmly for at least 2 minutes with the heel of your hand. A cursory rub for a few seconds won't do the trick, so keep going. This prevents the blood from blackening underneath the skin. Homoeopathic arnica reduces the negative effects of trauma and the likelihood of bruising 'coming out'. Rub arnica cream or arnica oil (from health stores and chemists) into the damaged area three times each day for two or three days afterwards. And take a vitamin C complex with bioflavonoids (1,000 mg three times daily).

☀ Burns

For serious burns, seek medical attention without delay.

For minor burns where the skin is unbroken: hold the burnt area under a cold tap or immerse in a bowl of iced water; keep immersed for as long as the pain continues.

Bach Rescue Remedy Cream or essential oil of lavender are soothing and healing to burned but unbroken skin. For me, one of the best soothers and healers is Aloe 99 Gel (Xynergy Health). I always keep a tube in my kitchen cupboard in case of burns or scalds.

Taking vitamins A, C and E and zinc internally should hasten the healing of burns.

If you have help at hand, this old remedy is confirmed by surgeons in Holland to be at least as good as current orthodox methods: cover the area with cooled (cleaned and boiled) potato peelings and wrap with sterilized cotton cloth or bandages. Change the peelings twice daily.

Chafing

Apricot and sesame seed oil are both excellent remedies for preventing the chafing caused by sports gear and new shoes. Cracked heels respond well to nightly massage with olive oil, cocoa butter or a nourishing foot cream.

Chapped Hands and Cracked Heels

Use a hand cream that contains vitamin E and/or aloe vera or add the contents of a vitamin E capsule or a dollop of Aloe 99 Gel to your own favourite hand cream and massage into your hands and feet, paying special attention to heels, nails and cuticles.

Wear protective gloves for household jobs and always protect hands with mitts or gloves in cold weather. Take GLA or evening primrose oil every day, especially throughout the winter months. Avoid sugar and sugary foods. Eat plenty of sunflower, pumpkin and linseeds and oily fish. Use cold-pressed oils for salad dressings and extra virgin olive oil for cooking.

Chilblains

Chilblains are an inflammation of the fingers or toes, usually due to poor a circulation and inadequate nutrition.

Take a regular vitamin C complex and a blood vessel-strengthener such as Biocare Beetroot Extract or an antioxidant with attitude such as Biocare Vitaflavan or the Solgar Proanthocyanidin Complex.

Freshly juiced raw beetroot is helpful for the blood and circulation too.

Eat more dark green vegetables and fresh fruits, live yoghurt, nuts and seeds.

Vitamin E (100–400 iu daily) and GLA or evening primrose oil capsules, taken with the evening meal, can be a wonderful boost to a sluggish circulation.

Homoeopathic silica is another useful remedy.

Massage painful chilblains with calendula or arnica cream.

✳ Cracked, Chapped Lips

Lips crack very easily because the skin covering them is very thin and has no moisturizing oil supply of its own.

Use Bach Rescue Remedy Cream daily under lipstick or by itself to lubricate dry lips and apply a protective coat of the same cream before bedtime. Other great soothers include Jurlique Lip Care Balm, Thursday Plantation Tea Tree LipGuard and Bioforce 7 Herb Cream.

When using facial scrubs, exfoliate gently over and around the lip area to remove any dead skin.

Troubled by cold sores? See page 220.

✳ Cuts

If the cut is deep, seek medical help.

Six drops of myrrh essential oil or tincture mixed well into warm water is a useful mixture for cleansing dirty wounds.

Superficial cuts will heal more quickly if bathed in aloe vera juice. Blot dry with a clean, lint-free cloth and then cover in Aloe 99 Gel. Allow the gel to dry and then apply a fresh dry sticking plaster if necessary. Re-apply Aloe 99 and change the dressing twice a day.

If water and towels are not available to clean the wound immediately, echinacea tincture, such as Bioforce Echinaforce, makes a good emergency wash. Simply hold the dropper over the wound and douse liberally.

Once a cut has closed up and is beginning to heal, rub it daily with the contents of a vitamin E capsule to prevent scarring.

Dry, Cracked, Chapped and Flaky Skin

Stuffy, overheated and air conditioned homes and offices and chilling outdoor winds can make skin dry, sore and prone to broken veins. Going in an out in extreme temperatures can do the same. So can over-exposure to drying summer wind and UV rays.

* Restore the skin's protective acid mantle by rinsing with organic cider vinegar, either diluted and splashed over the skin or applied with cotton wool.
* Watch out for sudden or frequent changes of temperature. In drying conditions moisture is lost from the skin faster than it can be replaced, so make regular daily use of the water-mist sprays mentioned on pages 204 and 217.
* Where broken thread veins are visible, massage the area very gently each night with the contents of a vitamin E capsule.
* Foods rich in flavonoids – and flavonoids supplements – are helpful for this condition. See page 44.
* Drink plenty of water throughout the day, winter and summer.
* Moisturize, moisturize, moisturize.

Herpes

Herpes is a highly contagious viral condition; once the virus has taken up residence in the body, it can lie dormant for years but will never go away.

However, if treated correctly it *is* controllable. There are many kinds of herpes, which fall into two distinct groups: *herpes simplex* and *herpes zoster*.

Herpes simplex is an inflammatory skin condition characterized by the formation of small clusters of watery blisters. Cold sores (*herpes labialis*) belong to this 'family', as does *herpes genitalis*, which affects the mucous membranes of the genitalia. Both are highly contagious and can be passed from one part of the body to another by touch. It is imperative to be cautious during an attack of herpes because of its contagiousness. The virus can be passed easily by kissing. This kind of herpes is a sexually-transmitted disease; intimate contact during an attack is obviously not recommended. Unfortunately, however, symptoms are not always visible and may take several weeks to appear – if at all. If you do suspect herpes infection, it is imperative that you see your GP without delay.

Herpes zoster (shingles) is an acute inflammatory condition triggered by the same virus that causes chicken-pox and which affects the nervous system. Pain during an attack can be very severe indeed and is often followed by a post-herpetic neuralgia.

Medical treatment of herpes with antiviral drugs can be very effective, but supporting the immune system and managing stress are two key factors in the control and prevention of herpes. Herpes is also believed to have a hormonal connection, since flare-ups do sometimes happen during periods.

Improving the quality of the diet and taking regular supplements can boost the immunity, strengthen stress-resistance and help to balance hormones.

I have found particular success by simply improving the nutritional quality of the diet, making sure it includes at least three portions of fresh vegetables, one big fresh salad and two or three pieces of fresh fruit daily. Also fresh fish, sunflower and pumpkin seeds, sheep's or goat's yoghurt and extra virgin olive oil, fresh vegetables and fruit juices and at least a litre of uncarbonated bottled or filtered water daily.

Herpes sufferers should avoid stimulants such as alcohol, salt, sugar, nicotine and caffeine, hydrogenated vegetable oil, and artificial food colourings, preservatives and flavourings.

If you have herpes and would like to try using nutritional supplements to ease your condition, these are the ones I have found most helpful with my own patients:

- ❋ A multivitamin/mineral complex which contains vitamins A, E, B_6 and zinc (one daily). Try Viridian, Biocare or Solgar.
- ❋ Vitamin B_{12} (injections once monthly for three months from your GP, or a once-daily, three-month supply of enteric-coated tablets [Biocare]). Vitamin B_{12} is the anti-pernicious anaemia vitamin but also has a major role to play in the function of a healthy nervous system, proving useful in the treatment of a range of neurological conditions.
- ❋ 2 grams of vitamin C complex daily. Vitamin C is naturally anti-viral, helps boost immunity and has natural painkilling activity.
- ❋ Free-form amino acid powders containing lysine, well known for the amelioration of herpes. This product is expensive and, in any event, *is best taken only under a practitioner's supervision*. More information from Biocare.
- ❋ *Lactobacillus acidophilus* probiotic supplements help to improve the quality of friendly bacteria in the gut and to boost immunity. In addition, probiotics have an oestrogen-balancing activity which may be a helpful addition in the treatment of herpes.
- ❋ Flavonoids, often included in good vitamin C supplements, help to reduce inflammation and are also powerful antioxidants. More on flavonoids on page 44.
- ❋ Vitamin E is useful for both topical and oral treatment of herpes. Take 300–400 iu twice daily with meals. In addition, apply the contents of one or two capsules to affected areas. Remember to wash the hands thoroughly after application. Vitamin E acts to reduce inflammation and, as a result, may also reduce pain. It has been used very successfully in the treatment of neuralgia pain associated with herpes zoster.

※ Tea tree oil is useful for many different skin problems including herpes, spots, insect bites and stings, sheep ticks, cuts, grazes, fungal infestations of the feet and nails, even head lice. Preparations containing essential oil of tea tree can be dabbed on to affected areas. Use a clean cotton bud or cotton pad for each application to prevent cross-infection.

If you're troubled by cold sores, I'd recommend Thursday Plantation Tea Tree Lip Fix and Bioforce Echinacea Cream.

Always wash the hands thoroughly after touching or treating any area of the body affected by herpes,

⁂ Itchy Skin

Try putting 1 tablespoon of extra virgin olive oil and 2 tablespoons of organic cider vinegar (not malt or wine vinegar) in the bath water. It helps to rebalance skin pH. Very soothing, too, for psoriasis, eczema and dermatitis and for that most embarrassing and distressing of 'itches', pruritis.

Chickweed cream – also sometimes sold under its Latin name *Stellaria* is an ancient herbal remedy much favoured by the Anglo-Saxon tribes which is still used today to treat rashes, urticaria and general skin irritation. Available from good herbal pharmacies such as Neal's Yard and Apotheke (see the Resources chapter for details).

Echinaforce Cream from Bioforce or any brand of good quality calendula cream such as Nelsons or Jurlique, will soothe itchy skin.

If skin is generally itchy all over but you can't seem to find the cause, suspect your washing powder, fabric softener, shampoo, soap, body lotion or shower gel. Go for a non-biological, phosphate-free liquid for your washing machine. Or try the eco-friendly Turbo Laundry Disc from Savant-Health or Eco-Balls from the Eco-Company, which clean without the use of detergents. Stockist info is on page 229. Change to hypoallergenic, preservative and perfume-free body care and hair products. There are plenty around. If possible, buy sample sizes first to see if they suit you. I've heard good reports of the Allergenics range of Gently Medicated Shampoo and Shower Gel, available from major chemists and most health stores. Stockist information is on page 229.

✻ Scarring

To reduce the risk of scars forming (after accident or surgery), as soon as stitches are removed rub the oil from a vitamin E capsule gently but firmly into the traumatized area every night before bedtime. The same method can help to fade old scars, too.

✻ Sore Eyes

Bathe with a very dilute Eyebright solution. The anti-inflammatory properties of Eyebright (Latin name *Euphrasia*) are helpful for all kinds of eye grittiness – and useful, too, for general tiredness of the eyes and where there is abnormal sensitivity to light.

- ✻ Swallow herbal Eyebright tablets or tincture; available from most health food stores. I use Euphrasian drops from Bioforce.
- ✻ Rest quietly in a darkened room with the eyes gently (not tightly) closed for 15 minutes during the day.
- ✻ Cold tea bags, squeezed out – one over each eye – reduce redness, puffiness and that gritty feeling.
- ✻ Take a best quality antioxidant complex (Biocare Cellguard Forte or Solgar Advanced Antioxidant Formula) daily.

✻ Sore Throats

At the very first sign of symptoms, start taking Echinaforce drops three times daily. A sore throat may be the first sign of a cold virus. Echinacea, especially if taken together with 2 or 3 grams of vitamin C and zinc lozenges, can knock a cold on the head before it gets hold of you.

For any kind of sore throat, try these gargles:

* 2 teaspoons of organic cider vinegar and 1 teaspoon of Comvita Manuka honey into a cup or mug; top up with boiling water and then wait for it to cool to a comfortable temperature.
* 6 drops of Comvita Propolis Extract dissolved in a glass of water.

Gargle until all the mixture has been used. Swallow each mouthful or spit it out. Repeat the process five or six times each day, but especially first thing in the morning and last thing at night. Continue with the gargle for a couple of days after symptoms have subsided. Use the whole drink at each session and make a fresh batch each time.

Spots and Pimples

Golden seal herbal infusion used as a skin rinse is soothing and healing.

Self-disinfecting 'spot' pens are also useful for emergency treatment, but beware of anti-spot treatments which have too strong an alcohol base as they can be harsh and over-drying. Those based on active essential oils seem to be the most successful. One of my favourite treatments is the Formule B Spotpen from Samuel Par, available in major Tesco outlets, Boots, independent chemists and health stores. Another is Blackmores Anti-Bacterial Pimple Gel. At the first sign of a spot, dab on the Gel or the Spotpen formula and repeat throughout the day. See also Samuel Par Nighshift (page 211). Most spots will fade very quickly if treated in this way.

Follow the dietary advice for spots – see page 140.

Sprains

To bring down swelling, make a cold compress with diluted witch hazel, cold used tea bags, or ice cubes.

Massage the affected area very gently with arnica or calendula ointment.

Take arnica tablets every two hours to ease shock and reduce the risk of bruising.

✳ Mouth Ulcers

✳ Improve the nutrient content of your diet. Increase intake of vegetables in the form of juices, soups and salads and eat more fresh fruit.

✳ Have a small carton of plain yoghurt (sheep's or goat's milk, not cow's milk) every day.

✳ Include daily supplements of B complex, zinc, vitamin A, beta carotene and liquorice.

✳ Change to a natural toothpaste. Try those from Blackmores, The Green People Company, Neal's Yard, Bioforce or Weleda.

✳ Sage and calendula or aloe vera mouthwash are soothing and healing.

✳ Tincture of myrrh is an effective remedy for dabbing directly on to mouth ulcers or for use as a mouthwash: add 3 ml of the tincture to a glass of water and use four times daily.

✳ Spread the contents of a vitamin E capsule onto the ulcerated area, after teeth cleaning, last thing at night.

Resources

Helpful Organizations

Colon Health

Colonic International Association
16 Englands Lane
London NW3 4TT
020 7483 1595

Eczema

The National Eczema Society
4 Tavistock Place
London WC1H 9RA

Food Allergy Testing

Allergycare
Pollards Yard, Wood Street
Taunton, Somerset TA1 1UP
01823 325023
Uses VEGA testing

Superskin

Apotheke Natural Health & Wellness Centre
296 Chiswick High Road
London W4 1PA
020 8995 2293
www.apotheke20-20.co.uk
A naturopathic and herbal clinic that uses the Bioenergetic Stress Testing System

British Society for Allergy and Environmental Medicine
P.O. Box 28
Totton
Southampton SO40 2ZA

ELISA Systems
01353 862220
www.hometest.co.uk
or
0800 074 6185
www.allergy.co.uk

The Hale Clinic
7 Park Crescent
London W1N 3HE
020 7631 6310
A number of different systems are available

Higher Nature Ltd
Burwash Common
East Sussex TN19 7LX
01435 883484

York Nutritional Laboratories
Murton Way
Osbaldwick
York YO19 5US

Herbalism

National Institutes of Medical Herbalists
56 Longbrook Street
Exeter
Devon EX4 6AH
01392 426022

General Council & Register of Consultant Herbalists
Grosvenor House
40 Sea Way
Middleton-on-Sea
West Sussex PO22 7BA

A-Z of Stockists

The following list contains contact details for the products and services
I've recommended in the book. It's not an exhaustive list, but does
include products that I've tried personally and would recommend. Some
are available by direct mail, others from health stores or pharmacies.
Contact individual companies for further information.

At-a-glance Products/Suppliers

Acidophilus probiotics	Biocare, Blackmores
Comvita cold-pressed honey	Health stores or contact New Zealand Natural Foods or Xynergy Health

Detergent-free washing discs	Eco-Co and Healthy House
Dr Bach Flower remedies	Health stores and chemists. Stockist information: 0800 289515
Essential fatty acids (evening primrose oil, GLA, etc.)	Arkopharma, Biocare, Pharma Nord, Solgar, Viridian Nutrition
Essential oils and atomizers	Absolute Aromas, Floressence, Gerard House, Jurlique, Neal's Yard, Nelsons, Passion for Life Products, Tisserand
Facial rejuvenator	Added Dimension Dentistry
Herbal remedies	Arkopharma, Bioforce, Bio-Health, The Green People Company, Viridian Nutrition
Juicing equipment	Most electrical retailers and houseware stores supply juicers (e.g. Magimix, Moulinex, Bosch, Braun, Kenwood). Green Power Juicer and Green Life Juicer are supplied by Savant. Magimix Le Duo is also available from Lakeland Ltd
Linseeds	GNC and other health stores stock Linusit Gold (stockist information 020 8477 5358); Linoforce linseeds are available from health stores, or contact Bioforce
Multivitamins and antioxidants	Biocare, Blackmores, Pharma Nord, Solgar, Viridian Nutrition
Natural-as-possible Skin and Hair care	Blackmores, Eco-Co, Felici, The Green People Company, Jurlique, Natracare, Neal's Yard, Passion for Life Products, Samuel Par (Formule B range)
Natural toothcare	Many health stores stock a wide range of excellent, chemical-free toothpastes,

	including Blackmores, Bioforce, The Green People Company and Weleda
Organic chocolate	Green & Black
Organic herbal and regular teas	Jurlique, Neal's Yard, Passion for Life, health stores and some supermarkets
Pure Aloe 99 gel	Xynergy Health
Spirulina/green juice	Naturopathic Health & Beauty Company, Xynergy Health
Vitamin E cream	Passion for Life Products, Xynergy Health

For contact details for these suppliers, see below.

Absolute Aromas
2 Grove Park
Mill Lane
Alton
Hampshire GU34 2QG
01420 549991
essential oils

Added Dimension Dentistry
First Floor
18 Wimpole Street
London W1M 7AD
020 7636 9978
www.newface.co.uk
ADD Facial Rejuvenator

Superskin

Biocare
180 Lifford Lane
Kings Norton
Birmingham B30 3NU
0121 433 3727
e-mail: sales@biocare.co.uk
multivitamins, minerals and antioxidants; essential fatty acids (evening primrose oil, GLA, etc.); acidophilus probiotics; herbals

Bioforce
2 Brewster Place
Irvine
Ayrshire KA11 5DD
01294 277344
www.bioforce.co.uk
herbal remedies (specializes in herbal tinctures including Violaforce and Echinaforce); Linoforce linseeds; Neem Hair Care

Bio-Health
Medway City Estate
Rochester
Kent ME2 4HU
01634 290115
herbal remedies

Blackmores UK
Willowtree Marina
West Quay Drive
Yeading
Middlesex UB4 9TB
020 8842 3956
multivitamins, minerals and antioxidants; herbs; acidophilus probiotics; natural-as-possible skin, body and hair care products

Eco-Co
Birchwood House
Briar Lane
Croydon
Surrey CRO 5AD
07071 223030
e-mail: info@eco-ball.co.uk
www.eco-co.co.uk
natural-as-possible skin and hair care products; Eco-balls and Eco-zyme cleaning products (re-usable detergent-free washing discs, recommended for anyone suffering eczema, allergies or dry skin conditions); wide range of eco-friendly skin care, body care, household products; vitamins and minerals; Green People Company and Biocare products.

Felici
Available from health stores, some beauty therapists or by mail order from
Natural Woman Ltd
86 Shirehampton Road
Stoke Bishop
Bristol BS9 2DR
0117 968 7744
www.natural-woman.com
natural-as-possible skin and hair care products

Floressence at Chamberlins
5 High Street
Waltham on the Wolds
Leicestershire LE14 4AH
01664 464468
e-mail: chamberlins@btinternet.com
essential oils

Superskin

Formule B
023 9244 9313
www.laformule.com
Formule B skin care for problem skins

Gerard House
Peter Black Healthcare
Consumer helpline: 01283 228344
essential oils; herbal medicines

Green and Black
Stockist information: 020 7243 0562
organic chocolate

The Green People Company
Brighton Road
Handcross
West Sussex RH17 6BZ
01444 401444
e-mail: info@greenpeople.co.uk
herbal remedies; natural-as-possible skin and hair care products; natural organic skin care suitable for dry, sensitive and irritated skin; also liquid soap, hand cream, hair care, toothpaste

Healthy House
Cold Harbour
Ruscombe
Stroud
Glos GL6 6DA
01453 752216
Fax: 01453.753533
www.healthy-house.co.uk

Eco-ball detergent-free washing discs and Eco-zyme cleaning products; anti-house dust mite bedding, organic cottons, filters, air purifiers, ionizers, emf protection, water purifiers, light boxes

Jurlique
see Naturopathic Health & Beauty
essential oils; atomizers (from the Naturopathic Health & Beauty Company); natural-as-possible skin and hair care products; organic herbal and regular teas

Natracare
From health stores, or by mail order from:
Natural Woman Ltd
86 Shirehampton Road
Stoke Bishop
Bristol BS9 2DR
0117 968 7744
www.natural-woman.com
natural-as-possible skin and hair care products including Natracare Baby Lotion and Barrier Cream

Naturopathic Health & Beauty Co
Postal address:
Willowtree Marina
West Quay Drive
Yeading
Middlesex UB4 9TB
020 8841 6644
Jurlique and Blackmores products; spirulina/green juice (Hawaiian Pacifica Organic Spirulina); skin care and hair care products; essential oils

Neal's Yard Remedies

0161 831 7875

www.nealsyardremedies.com

e-mail: mail@nealsyardremedies.com

essential oils and atomizers, floral waters; natural-as-possible skin and hair care products; organic herbal and regular teas; herbal, homoeopathic remedies

Nelson & Russell

For stockist information call 020 7495 2404

essential oils

New Zealand Natural Foods

55–7 Park Royal Road

London NW10 7LP

020 8961 4410

www.nznf.co.uk

e-mail: info@xynergy.co.uk

Manuka products; best quality organic honey; Comvita cold-pressed honey; Comvita propolis range

Passion for Life Products Ltd

Grove House

320 Kensal Road

London W10 5BZ

0800 096 1121 (UK only)

+44 208 964 9944 (international)

www.passionforlife.com

e-mail: info@passionforlife.com

essential oils; vitamin E cream; natural-as-possible skin and hair care products; organic herbal and regular teas

Saguna Silicol Skin gel
08707 274153

Samuel Par
02392 449314
www.samuelpar.co.uk
natural-as-possible skin and hair care products (Formule B range)

Savant-Health
15 Iveson Approach
Leeds
West Yorkshire LS16 6LJ
0113 230 1993
www.savant-health.com
e-mail: savant@mail.com
Turbo Plus Ceramic Laundry Disc; organic linseed oil; juicing machines

The Soil Association
If you have access to the Internet, why not visit the excellent Soil Association website at www.soilassociation.org. Or write to them for regional guides on where to find organics at:
Bristol House
40–56 Victoria Street
Bristol BS1 6BY
Don't forget to enclose a large stamped addressed envelope.

AUTHOR'S NOTE
I'd like to express my grateful thanks to the Soil Association for the information they have provided for the chapter on Organics.

Superskin

Thursday Plantation
01274 488511
www.teatree.co.uk
tea tree products, also available from good health stores

Viridian Nutrition
31 Alvis Way
Daventry
Northamptonshire NN11 5PG
01327 878050
Fax/ansaphone: 01327 878335
www.viridian-nutrition.com
multivitamins, minerals and antioxidants; essential fatty acids (evening primrose oil, GLA, etc.); herbal supplements
Viridian Nutrition donates a significant proportion of its net profits to charity.

Xynergy Health
Elstead, Midhurst
West Sussex GU29 0JT
01730 813642
Fax: 01739 815109
www.xynergy.co.uk
Pure Aloe 99 Gel; Aloe 99 vitamin E cream, biogenic aloe vera juice, Comvita propolis products; Comvita Manuka cold-pressed honey; spirulina/ green juice (Pure Synergy)

Recommended Reading

The Inside Story
Berrydales Publishers
Berrydale House
5 Lawn Road
London NW3 2XS
Highly recommended newsletter for allergy sufferers. Please send s.a.e. for subscription details.

What Doctors Don't Tell You and *Proof!*
If health matters to you, I would highly recommend a regular subscription to one or both of these excellent journals.
Send an s.a.e. to:
Wallace Press
Satellite House
2 Salisbury Road
London SW19 4EZ
www.wddty.co.uk
e-mail: info@wddty.co.uk
Back issues of *Psoriasis – Chemical Overkill* are available from the *What Doctor's Don't Tell You* publishers for £4.95 including postage. Ask for Volume 4, Issue number 3.

References

Superskin Foods and the Importance of Fats

5th International Colloquium on Monounsaturated Fatty Acids. 17 and 18 February 1992.

Isles C.G., Hole D.J., Gillis C.R. et al., "Plasma cholesterol, coronary heart disease and cancer". *Br.Med.J.* 1989; 298:920–24.

Dietary Reference Values for Food Energy and Nutrients for the United Kingdom. Report of the Panel on Dietary Reference Values of the Committee on Medical Aspects of Food Policy.

Mensink R.P., Katan M.B., "Effect of a diet enriched with monounsaturated or polyunsaturated fatty acids on levels of low-density lipoprotein cholesterol in healthy men and women". *N.Eng.J.Med.* 1989; 321(7):436–41.

Holborow P., "Melanoma patients consume more polyunsaturated fat than people without melanoma". *N.Z. Med.J.* 27.11.91 p.502.

McMichael, Sir J., report in *Br.Med.J.* January 1979.

Halliwell B., *Free Radicals and Food Additives*, Taylor & Francis, 1991.

Brisson Professor G.J., *Lipids in Human Nutrition*.

Williams Dr Roger, *Nutrition Against Disease*.

Antioxidant Vitamins and Beta Carotene in Disease Prevention International Conference. October 1989.

Clausen J., Nielsen S.A., Kristensen M., "Biochemical and clinical effects of an antioxidative supplementation of geriatric patients". *Biological Trace Element Research* 1989; 20:135–51.

Chow G.K., "Nutritional influence on cellular antioxidant defence systems". *American Journal of Clinical Nutrition* 1979; 32:1066–81.

Gutteridge J.M., Westermarck T., Halliwell B., "Oxygen radical damage in biological systems". *Free Radicals, Ageing and Degenerative Disease* 1986; pp.99–139.

Ito N., Hirose M., *Antioxidants – carcinogenic and chemopreventive properties* 1989; 53:247–302.

Vital Skin Nutrients

Cheraskin E., *Vitamin C – Who needs it?*, Arlington Press, 1993.

Gaby A., "Natural remedies and the drug cartel: The use of bioflavonoids to treat hemorrhagic purpura", *Literature Commentary and Review* April 1992: 226.

Havsteen B., "Flavonoids – a class of natural products of high pharmaceutical potency", *Biochemistry and Pharmacology* 1983, 32: 1141–8.

Knek E.P. et al., "Flavonoid intake and coronary mortality in Finland", *British Medical Journal* 1996, 312: 478–81.

Masquier J., "Pycnogels: Recent advantages in the therapeutic activity of procyanidins", *Journal of Medicinal Plant Research* 1980, 7: 243–56.

Mervyn L., "The extraordinary properties of pine bark extract", Undated copy article.

Middleton E., "Some biological properties of plant flavonoids", *Annals of Allergy* 1988, 61 [2]: 53–7.

Middleton E. et al., "Naturally occurring flavonoids and human basophil histamine release", *Archives of Allergy and Applied Immunology* 1985, 77: 155–7.

Muldoon M.F. et al., "Flavonoids and heart disease", *British Medical Journal* 1996, 312: 458–9.

Pauling L. and Rath M., "An orthomolecular theory of human health and disease", *Journal of Orthomolecular Medicine* 1991, 6: 135–8

Picq M. et al., "Effects of two flavonoid compounds on central nervous system", *Life Sciences* 1991, 49: 1979–88

De Whalley C.V. et al., "Flavonoids inhibit the oxidative modification of low-density lipoprotein cholesterol", *Biochemistry and Pharmacology* 1990, 39: 1743–9.

Okita M. et al., "Lipid malnutrition of patients with liver cirrhosis; effect of low intake of dietary lipid on plasma fatty acid composition" *Acta Med Okayama* 1989; 43:39–45.

Zurer B., "Essential fatty acids and inflammation". Ann Rheum Dis. 1991; 50:745–46.

Holborow P., "Melanoma and fatty acids". *NZ Med.J.* 1991; 104:19.

Begin M. et al., "Plasma fatty acid levels in patients with Acquired Immune Deficiency Syndrome and in controls". *Prostaglandins Leukotr EFAs* 1989; 37:135–37.

Williams L.L. et al., "Serum fatty acid composition of plasma from MDS patients and normal individuals". *Arch AIDS RES.* 1988; 23:981–88.

Manku M., Horrobin D.E, Morse N.L. et al., "Essential fatty acids in the plasma phospholipids of patients with atopic eczema". *Br J Dermatol.* 1984; 110:643–48.

Horrobin D.F., "Essential fatty acids, immunity and viral infections". *J Nutr Med.* 1990; 1:145–51.

Horrobin D.F., "Essential fatty acids and the post-viral fatigue syndrome" Book: *Post Viral Fatigue Syndrome*, Ed. Jenkins R. and Mowbray J. John Wiley, Chichester and New York, 1991.

Wolfe S.M., *Pills That Don't Work*, pp. 1819. Public Citizen Research Group.

Colbin A., *Food and Healing*, pp. 15–23, Ballantine Books.

Medawar C., *The Wrong Kind of Medicine*, Consumers' Association/ Hodder & Stoughton, August 1984.

Coutsoudis A., Coovadia H.M., Broughton M., Salisbury R.T., Elson I., "Micronutrient utilization during measles treated with vitamin A or placebo". *Int J Vitamin Nutrition Review* 1991; 61:199–204.

Daulaire N. et al., "Childhood mortality after a high dose of vitamin A in a high risk population". *Br.Med.J.* 1992; 304:207–10.

Zile M.H., Cullum M.E., "The function of vitamin A – current concepts". *Proceedings of the Society of Experimental Biological Medicine* 1983; 172:139–52.

Horwitt M.K., "Data supporting supplementation of humans with vitamin E". *J Nutr.* 1991; 121:424–29.

Janero D.R., "Therapeutic potential of vitamin E in the pathogenesis of spontaneous atherosclerosis". *Free Radical Biology & Medicine* 1991; 11:129–44.

Marsden K., "Vitamin C, the master nutrient versus heart disease, the master killer". (article) *Int. J. Alt. Comp. Med.* October 1992 pp. 19–20.

Pauling L., Rath M., "Solution to the puzzle of human cardiovascular disease". *J Orthomolecular Med.* 1991; 6:125–34.

Ginter E., "Vitamin C deficiency, cholesterol metabolism and atherosclerosis". *J Orthomolecular Med.* 1991: 6:166–72.

Goodman, S., *Vitamin C – The Master Nutrient*, Keats Publishing Inc.

Ginter E., Bobek P., Kubec F., Vozar J., Urbanova D., "Vitamin C in the control of hypercholesterolaemia in man". *International Journal of Vitamin and Nutritional Research* 1982; 23:137–52.

Gorrie D.R., "Purpura haemorrhagica after arsenic therapy treated by vitamin P". *Lancet* 1940; 1:1005–7.

Middleton E. et al., "Natually occurring flavonoids and human basophil histamine release". *Archives of Allergy & Applied Immunology* 1985; 77:155–57.

Rixier J.M., Godeau G., Robert A.M. and Hornebeck W., "In vivo and in vitro study demonstrating that binding of Pycnogenol to elastin affects its rate of degradation". *Biochem.Pharmacol.* 1984; 33(24):3933–39.

Havsteen B., "Flavonoids, a class of natural products of high pharmaco-logical potency". Article. *Biochem.Pharmacol.* 1983; 32(7):1141–48.

Ginter E., "Vitamin C deficiency, cholesterol metabolism and atheroscle-rosis". *J Orthomolecular Med.* 1991; 6:166–72.

Roediger W.E.W., Lawson M.J., Radcliffe B.C., "Nitrite from inflamma-tory cells – a cancer risk factor in ulcerative colitis?" *Dis Colon Rectum.* 1990; 33:1034–36.

Tanji J.L., "Dietary calcium as a treatment for mild hypertension". *J Amer Board Family Practice* 1991; 4:145–50.

Lipkin M., "Calcium, vitamin D and colon cancer". *Cancer Res.* 1991; 51:3069–70.

Bachert C. et al., "Decreased reactivity in allergic rhinitis after intra-venous application of calcium. A study on the alteration of local airway resistance after nasal allergen provocation". *Arzneimittelforsch.* (trans-lation) 1990; 40:984–87.

Anderson R.A. et al., "Supplemental chromium effects on glucose, insulin, glucagon and urinary chromium losses in subjects consuming low chromium diets". *Am J Clin Nutr.* 1991; 54:909–16.

Roeback J., "Effect of chromium supplementation on serum high-density lipoprotein cholesterol levels in men taking beta-blockers". *Ann Int Med.* 1991; 115(12):917–24.

Barber S.A., Bull N.L. and Buss D.H., "Low Iron Intake Among Young Women in Britain." *Br.Med.J.* 1985; 290:743–44.

Woods K.L., Fletcher S., Roffe C, Haider Y., "Intravenous magnesium sulphate in suspected acute myocardial infarction: results of second Leicester Intravenous Magnesium Intervention Trial". *Lancet* 1992; 39:1553–58.

Facchinetti F. et al., "Oral magnesium successfully relieves premenstrual mood changes". *Obstet Gyn.* 1991; 78:177–81.

Peretz A. et al., "Adjuvant treatment of recent onset rheumatoid arthritis by selenium supplementation". *Br J Rheumatal.* 1992; 31:281–86.

Abraham G.E., "The importance of magnesium in the management of pri-mary osteoporosis". *J Nutr Med.* 1991; 2:165–78.

Acne, Eczema and Psoriasis

Bassett I.B., Pannowitz D.L and Barnetson R.S.C., "A comparative study of tea-tree oil versus benzoyl peroxide in the treatment of acne". *Med.J.Australia* 1990; 153:455–58.

Manku M.S., Horrobin D.E, Morse N.L., Wright S. and Burton J.L., "Essential fatty acids in the plasma phospholipids of patients with atopic eczema". *British Journal of Dermatology* 1984; 110:643–48.

Ziboh V.A. and Chapkin R.S., "Metabolism and function of skin lipids". *Progress in Lipid Research* 1988; 27:81–105.

Burton J.L., "Dietary fatty acids and inflammatory skin disease". *Lancet* 7.1.89; 27–30.

Lewis Jenny, *The Eczema Handbook*, Vermilion.

___, *The Psoriasis Handbook*, Vermilion.

Vahlquist C. et al., "The fatty acid spectrum in plasma and adipose tissue in patients with psoriasis". *Archives of Dermatological Research* 1985; 278:114–19.

Maurice P. et al., "The effects of dietary supplementation with fish oil in patients with psoriasis". *British Journal of Dermatology* 1987; 177:599–606.

Stewart J.C., "Treatment of severe and moderately severe atopic dermatitis with evening primrose oil". *Journal of Nutritional Medicine* 1991; 2:9–15.

Sampson H., "Role of immediate food hypersensitivity in the pathogenesis of atopic dermatitis". *J. Allergy Clin. Immunology* 1983; 71:473–80.

Amella M. et al. "Inhibition of mast cell histamine release by flavonoids and bioflavonoids". *Planta Medica* 1985; 51:16–20.

Sleep

Penland J. "Effects of trace element nutrition on sleep patterns in adult women". *Federation of America Society of Experimental Biology Journal* 1988; 2:434.

Get Moving!

McGuire R., "Twice daily exercise may reduce hypertension". *Medical Tribune* 27 June 1991.

Blair S.N., Goodyear N.N., Gibbons L.W. et al., "Physical fitness and incidence of hypertension in healthy normotensive men and women". *Ann.Rev.Public Health* 1987; 252:480–87.

Leon A.S., Connett J., Jacobs D.R. et al., "Leisure time physical activity levels and risk of coronary heart disease and death. The Multiple Risk Factor International Trial". *J.Am.Med.Assoc.* 1987; 258:2388–95.

Duncan J.J. et al., "Women Walking For Health And Fitness: How Much Is Enough?" *J.Am.Med.Assoc.* 1991; 266 (23):3295–99.

Frankel T., "Walking may protect hips". *Prevention magazine* 8 February 1990.

Lennox S.S., Bedell F.R., Stone A.A., "The effect of exercise on normal mood". *J.Psychosomatic Res.* 1990; 34(6):629–636.

Braverman E.R., "Sports and Exercise: Nutritional Augmentation and Health Benefits". *J.Orthom.Med.* 1991; 6:191–201.

Caren L.D., "Effects of exercise on the human immune system: does exercise influence susceptibility to infections?" *Bioscience* 1991; 41:410–15.

McLellan R., Article on rebounding. *The American Chiropractor* June 1991, pp.10–14.

Index